HONG KONG REFLECTIONS

Hong Kong Reflections

Health, Illness and Disability in Hong Kong Children

David P. Davies

The Chinese University Press

ISBN 962–201–660–X

THE CHINESE UNIVERSITY PRESS
The Chinese University of Hong Kong
Sha Tin, New Territories
Hong Kong

Printed in Hong Kong by Nam Fung Printing Co., Ltd.

Contents

Prologue

My time as paediatrician in Hong Kong and Foundation Professor and Chairman of the Department of Paediatrics at The Chinese University of Hong Kong from my arrival in August 1982 until I left in July 1989, provided me with many opportunities to write on a wide range of topics of particular relevance to children in Hong Kong. Some contributions were on themes related to my particular clinical and research interests — growth and nutrition in early childhood and undergraduate education. Some I happened to become involved in more by accident than intention. Others were prompted by particular personal experiences. The present small anthology brings together fourteen of these contributions. They appear by kind permission of the editors of the various journals in which they were originally published. My Epilogue describes some final impressions on the variations in paediatric conditions between Hong Kong and Britain.

Historical appreciations are important in the development of any subject, expressing not only the culmination of past events and experiences but providing also foundations for future research and development. They reflect earlier successes and failures; they reflect narrow thinking and expansive ideals. In reading these chapters, I hope future paediatricians will obtain a glimpse of how some of the health problems of children in Hong Kong were thought of in the 1980s. Indeed, I would like to think that, in a small way, this volume complements that outstanding epidemiological study of health, growth and nutrition of Hong Kong infants and children in the 1960s, *Growing Up in Hong Kong* by Professor Elaine Field and Dr. Flora Baber from the University of Hong Kong, and to which frequent reference is made in some of my articles. What a significant historical pause this work provided, describing vividly the harrowing living environment of children in Hong Kong a generation ago and the effects of this on their health and development. Anyone who doubts the enormous advances that have been made in child health in Hong Kong in recent decades should read some of my contributions alongside that of Professor Field and Dr. Baber.

My time in Hong Kong, a short seven years, was memorable. Kindness, generosity and tolerance were always forthcoming. It is to my many friends and professional colleagues in Hong Kong, not forgetting the many medical students who passed through my hands, that I offer this anthology.

David P. Davies
May 1995

Part One

Growth and Nutrition

1

*Harmony and Discord**

The Hong Kong Journal of Paediatrics, 1985; 2:245–59

The word *growth* carries many varied connotations to different people. For parents, it immediately brings to mind increase in physical size of their children. For the embryologist, it will strike the chord of differential change in shape and size of the fetus early in development. For the physiologist, the emphasis might be more on functional events which underlie growth processes. For the biochemist, the interest is in the interactions between these metabolic processes. To the paediatrician, growth means one and all of these impressions, since knowledge of how a child grows and develops provides the scientific basis of paediatric practice.

In a biological context, the ultimate purpose behind the highly complex, yet remarkably orderly, scheme of growth and development of any organism (and in this the young human is no exception) is to achieve sexual maturity, thereby ensuring the potential for continued survival of the species. A child's growth and development can be likened to a journey, its many stages merging imperceptibly with each other. In this lecture, I would like you to travel this journey with me. In most instances it proceeds harmoniously, avoiding or mastering many potential obstacles on the way; on occasions, however, the journey is dark, distorted and tortuous with resulting discords striking alarming dissonance and responsible for much human misery.

The start of the journey is not birth but conception, forty weeks or so

* An inaugural lecture from the chair of Paediatrics delivered on 30 March 1984; reprinted with the permission of The Chinese University of Hong Kong.

earlier. Thereafter it unfolds through prenatal into postnatal life to reach its climax at adolescence. Life then enters a long period of decline into degeneration and decay! Birth intervenes early in this scheme. Momentous an event though it is, especially in regard to changes which have to take place in cardiorespiratory and gastrointestinal function, not to mention its immense social upheaval, the growth programme itself is little affected by birth. As Scammon has so aptly put it, "Birth marks not a beginning but a stage in life's journey."

Harmony: Some General Concepts

To set the scene for this eventful journey, I would like first to consider some important background features — fundamental physiological concepts of growth and its control. Without this appreciation, the purpose and the direction of the journey cannot be fully understood.

Organization of Growth Process

The basic unit of physical change which underlies increases in size, and its associated changing function, is cell growth, which through complex sequences of cell multiplication (hyperplasia) and increase in size (hypertrophy), though still poorly understood, lead to final mature structure. Normal physical growth of the body is the outward expression of harmonious increases in size of its organs and tissues which emerge differentiated out of the embryonic period. There are many fascinating aspects underlying the organization of growth and I would like to mention briefly two, chosen because of their particular relevance to clinical practice.

Brain Growth

The brain undergoes its period of most rapid growth before the rest of the body. One direct consequence of this sequence is that development, the physiological accompaniment of increase in size, must inevitably proceed in a cranio-caudal direction. This is how, for example, a young baby is first able to control the movements of its head before it begins the exploration of its environment. Interference with this normal process is all too readily obvious in the child whose brain has been damaged early in development. Furthermore, for the body to grow to its maximum potential, the brain has first to undergo normal growth. The brain therefore holds a key role in the control of the growth programme and development, although how this is mediated is not understood.

There are three principal phases of brain growth. In the first, completed by about twenty weeks of gestation, the neuronal cell complement is almost totally accomplished. The second phase, termed the principal brain growth spurt, begins at about twenty weeks of gestation, reaching a peak velocity at about forty weeks and is completed in about the fifth year after conception. This spurt initially involves a massive increase in the number of glial cells, a supporting cellular network which later takes on the role of laying down myelin sheaths around the axons of neurones and which also serve as a vital link in the chain by which neurones obtain their nutrition. Contemporaneously, the dense interlocking lattice of connections between the earlier formed neurones are also rapidly developing. The final phase of brain growth, which occupies the remainder of childhood and extends beyond the achievement of physical maturity, involves the elaboration of the incredibly intricate system of inter-neuronal connections, which probably lays the foundations for higher intellectual function.

This pattern of brain growth, which results in the brain at birth being already 25% and by the age of four about 75% of its adult weight, is far from being of simple academic curiosity. Vulnerability of the growth of any organ or tissue to environmental hazards is greatest when its growth is proceeding most rapidly. For the young human being, the greatest hazard is lack of food — both before and especially after birth. The implications for the many millions of children in the world who live in appalling conditions of endemic malnutrition before as well as after birth are abundantly clear. The apparently large heads of these deprived children is but an illusion. Their brains are already a distortion of their true genetic-potential from early interference and studies are beginning to indicate that, in addition to short-term physical toll of malnutrition, adverse long-term consequences to learning and behaviour also exist, as have been demonstrated previously from studies in experimental animals.

Growth of the Skeleton

The way in which the skeleton grows in length, and on which body stature largely depends, is somewhat different from the growth of the body organs where increase in size is due to increase in number and size of its cells. It takes place through the activity in the long bones and vertebrae of the growth plate, a zone of dividing cartilage cells separating the primary from the secondary ossification centres which subsequently lay down intercellular substances containing mineral salts surrounding the cells to form bone matrix. As the rate of growth slows down, the growth plate becomes narrower until eventually the bone in the main shaft joins with the bone in the epiphysis, thereby eliminating the growth plate. No further growth is possible, the epiphysis being "closed." At the same time as bone growth takes place, constant remodelling and moulding also occur in order to sustain the constant demands of subtle changes of shape taking place in the skeleton.

Control of Growth

How is growth, this most fundamental of body processes, controlled? It would be an understatement to say that much remains to be learned. Indeed, we know more about why growth does not take place than how it does. That the template for normal growth is contained in the individuals' genetic make-up is beyond dispute, with the genetic message being coded in many genes on many chromosomes. But how is this message transcribed into actual growth? For its optimum expression we do know that there must operate the appropriate milieu for growing organs and tissues. Of the endocrine secretions, those which are most important are *growth hormone*, synthesized in the anterior pituitary gland and which acts indirectly through another hormone elaborated in the liver, *somatomedin*, on the growing cells of the cartilage growth plate and muscle; *thyroid hormones* which are responsible for cell differentiation and protein synthesis in the nervous system, mitotic activity of the growth plate and maturation of ossification centres; and *androgens* (secreted by the adrenal gland) and the sex hormones, *testosterone* and *oestrogen*, which all contribute significantly to the puberty growth spurt in boys and girls.

These hormones can be considered as leaders of sections of an orchestra. Their conductor resides in the hypothalamus and higher centres of the brain. The actual playing at cellular level is mediated by a combination of hormones with receptor protein molecules in membranes of their target cells. These reactions cause an intracellular messenger to be released which speeds up certain intracellular mechanisms which ultimately cause an increase in size. Yet, in the absence of these hormones, growth will not cease but instead simply continue at a much slower rate. For example, children who lack growth hormone from the pituitary gland will still reach a size of 130 cm at maturity. Another intriguing fact is that hormones exert a far greater influence on growth after birth than during prenatal life. It is difficult therefore to escape the conclusion that growth contains an intrinsic momentum which is impossible to completely dampen. The mystery is, where does this intrinsic momentum come from: the composer remains anonymous! The following poem by Jon Ruhrah (1872) aptly describes our current predicament:

> We have the baby weighed today
> The nursing time is set
> At last we find we are so wise
> We can begin to standardise
> No baby now need fret
> In spite of this the baby grows
> But why it does — God only knows.

Stages of Growth

So much for the background of the journey. I would now like to consider its individual stages. These can be conveniently considered to take place in six periods, each with its own distinctive characteristics.

Before birth
Embryonic: Conception to 12 weeks
Early fetal: 12 to 28 weeks
Late fetal: 28 weeks to birth

After birth
Infancy: Birth to 18 months
Childhood: 18 months to 10–14 years
Adolescence: 10–14 years to 18–21 years

Growth before Birth

Embryonic

This is the period which is traditionally considered to extend from conception to about 12 weeks, and when the basic structure of the organs and tissues of the body becomes differentiated out of the three germ layers which have emerged in the early weeks following conception. The fetus enters the embryonic period a primitive being, unrecognizable as human: it emerges more easily recognizable as a member of *Homo sapiens* with arms and legs that move; a heart that beats; a nervous system that is beginning to show reflex activities; lungs beginning to rehearse breathing movements; and kidneys to produce urine. The understanding and study of these remarkably complex series of events that underlie this transfiguration are embraced by the science of embryology. Discord, as we will see later, arising during this period of embryogenesis can result in serious errors of morphogenesis (congenital malformations), the consequences of which have particular relevance to the paediatrician and a source of much human misery.

Early Fetal

This second stage extends to about 28 weeks — the upper limit of legally accepted viability. With improvements in the care of the fetus and new-born baby, the definition of viability is now in desperate need of revision. Many reports now point towards babies born between 23 and 28 weeks of gestation surviving. Indeed the social, moral, religious and medical consequences of what can be achieved through the harnessing of modern technology by ever-increasing clinical competence is disconcerting. This period of early fetal development witnesses the very rapid growth of the body. At 12 weeks, crown-rump length averages 8 cm and weight 50 g. At 28 weeks, these measures are 28 cm and 1,000 g respectively. Accompanying this huge increase in size are profound changes in external form in which, if there was doubt before, there can now be no doubt at all of the human characteristics of the developing organism — the fetus coming to look like a wizened old man, an appearance due mainly to an almost total absence of fat in the subcutaneous tissue.

Late Fetal

The early fetal period merges imperceptibly into the late fetal period. At 28 weeks, average body weight is about 1,000 g; at 40 weeks, it is around 3,000 g. The most obvious changes in appearance relate to fatness. Little fat is laid down early in pregnancy except for the structural phospholipids of cell membranes. Up to 20 weeks, only about 1% of body weight is made up of fat. During the second half of gestation, however, white fat, derived from transplacental glucose and fatty acid precursors, is rapidly laid down in specialized connective tissue cells in the skin and surrounding the internal organs, especially the kidney. As a result of these physiological processes, at 26 weeks the fetus has 2–3% fat in its body; at 35 weeks 8% and in a full-term baby of 3.5 kg about 15%. Of this, 80% is subcutaneous tissue and provides, along with valuable thermal insulation, an important energy store to cover the period immediately after birth when feeding is becoming established.

A detailed knowledge and understanding of prenatal human growth and development in this latter part of the fetal period has over the past couple of decades become increasingly important to the clinician. About 10% of babies at birth will show some type of growth disorder (to a greater or lesser extent) so as to expose them to perinatal risk. For the obstetrician, the serial measurement by ultrasound of certain fetal dimensions (e.g. the bi-parietal diameter of the head) has become an essential tool to monitor the physical well-being of the fetus, analogous in many ways to infancy and childhood where assessment of growth is also an essential cornerstone to evaluate well-being. Indeed, it is somewhat humbling to recall that until ultrasound was routinely introduced into clinical practice (about 15 to 20 years ago), physical growth of the fetus could be determined only by palpating the mother's abdomen at regular intervals. For the paediatrician, understanding how the fetus grows in latter part of pregnancy (knowledge of which has been built up primarily from measurements of the physical dimensions of weight, length and head circumference of babies born after varying lengths of gestation) provides a sound basis to assess the growth of not only infants who are born early in the third trimester and who, through improved neonatal care, now stand a much improved chance of survival, but also those born at term who demonstrate some anomaly of growth.

The rate of intra-uterine growth depends upon the extent to which the genetic growth potential of the fetus is allowed optimal expression by its immediate intra-uterine environment which in turn depends on (1) the mother, who, through her circulation, supplies essential nutrients and oxygen to the intervillous spaces of placenta, and (2) the placenta, itself a fetal organ, which exchanges nutrients and waste products between fetal and maternal circulation. Collectively these components can be considered the growth support or supply line of the fetus. It is interesting however to reflect that size at birth is often not a true reflection of genetic endowment for growth, even under physiological conditions. Since Walton and Hammond's studies in the 1930s of reciprocal crossings between Shire horses and Shetland ponies which first described a strong maternal influence on prenatal growth, many studies have consistently been able to demonstrate a profound maternal influence on total body growth, especially in its constraint where the fetus is destined to be bigger than the mother might be able to accommodate. Indeed, it has been estimated that only about 40% of birthweight variation can be attributed to genetic factors, the remaining 60% coming from the immediate environment of the fetus which in turn is largely influenced by the size and nutritional state of the mother. The contribution made by the father to the intra-uterine growth rate seems to be restricted to the donation of his genes to the conceptus. Birth provides the baby with a release from the shackles of maternal domination, allowing the baby to follow thereafter its own genetically determined direction.

Physiological Changes Accompanying Prenatal Growth

At this stage, I would like to pause on the journey to draw attention to some important aspects of physiological changes which accompany prenatal growth. These have, as their short-term objective, the preparation of the fetus for the difficult transition which lies ahead at birth when its environment is suddenly changed, forcing it to exchange its sheltered aquatic intra-uterine existence for a terrestrial one far more hostile. The essential body functions which must be established at birth and which are being prepared before birth are those performed in fetal life by the placental supply line to which I have earlier alluded to. They include especially: respiration, nutrition, maintenance of the *milieu interieur*, maintenance of body temperature, and protection against infection.

For as long as birth occurs at around the expected time, the functional changes which have taken place in the prenatal baby should have reached such a maturity as to allow in most instances, providing there are no environmental hazards, a smooth and efficient adaptation to the extra-uterine environment. Premature delivery, which occurs in about 6% of births in developed countries (but with often an almost threefold increased prevalence in underprivileged areas of the world), renders the new-born baby especially vulnerable, the extent of this physiological vulnerability being proportional to the degree of prematurity. Irregular control of breathing (respiratory centre immaturity), the need to feed milk into the stomach by feeding tube (due to immature sucking and swallowing mechanisms), jaundice (immaturity of enzyme activity in the liver), hypothermia (little fat to generate heat and provide thermal insulation) are commonly encountered problems. However, the most threatening problem results from the lack of surface active lipoproteins in the lungs which leads to difficulties in breathing and impaired exchange of oxygen and carbon dioxide — the syndrome of *hyaline membrane disease* which in severe cases will require assisted ventilation and is responsible for about one half of infant deaths in the early weeks after birth. Indeed, it is not sufficiently well appreciated that hyaline membrane disease is the single most common cause of death in childhood accounting for between 10% and 15% of all deaths under the age of 16 in the developed world. Under the age of 40, it is, next to accidents, the second most common cause of death. It is the attempt to manage the complex physiological consequences of this disorder that has been mostly responsible for the emergence over the last couple of decades of the discipline of neonatal intensive care. So successful has this become (under optimum practising conditions) that in babies of 1–1.5 kg at birth (28 to 32 weeks of gestation) who are born without major errors of morphogenesis, survival can be in the order of 95%. In the most technologically sophisticated units of the world, in babies born between 24 and 28 weeks — legally non-viable you will recollect — survival rates of up to 50% can be achieved. Regrettably, this survival is sometimes bought at a cost with tremendous human consequences — that of neuro-developmental handicap (cerebral palsy) as a consequence of structural brain damage caused by harmful influences such as lack of oxygen and haemorrhage which are the direct consequence of respiratory insufficiency.

Growth after Birth

Infancy and Childhood

So much for the first section of journey — the prenatal period — the part largely hidden from view. We now emerge from the foliage into an open plain where all aspects of growth can be more plainly seen. In day-to-day clinical practice, this part of the journey can be represented by the curve of growth.

The growth curve The growth curve in an individual child may be constructed from measurements such as height and weight taken at frequent intervals. It was a French naturalist, Count Philibert Guenau de Montbeillard, in the eighteenth century who was the first to collect a complete set of longitudinal height data from measurements in his own son taken every six months from birth to the age of 18. I use his data to describe the principal features. At any one time the journey can be described in terms of distance travelled (attained size) and the speed of travel (rate [velocity] of growth). Of these two measurements, the rate of growth is the more sensitive measure of current growth performance: attained size reflects far more previous experiences. When growth curves are constructed from measurements of large numbers of children, they provide the basis for standards to judge the growth performance of individual children.

Examination of this velocity curve of height reveals four well-defined phases. The first extends from the time the new-born infant has recovered from the terminal intra-uterine slowing of growth (between one and three weeks) and lasts until the age of about two. The prominent feature of this period is a steady deceleration in growth rate which has in fact been operating since about the thirtieth week of gestation. The second phase is characterized by much slower deceleration (which in actual practice is taken as an almost constant rate of growth) which lasts about ten years until the onset of the third phase — the adolescent growth spurt. When this is complete the child enters the fourth and final phase, that of growth deceleration, until, at maturity, growth in height ceases. A striking feature of the human growth curve is the long pre-adolescent phase, a phenomenon peculiar to primates and which reaches its maximum expression in the human. This long period of relative quiescence might teleologically be seen as providing the brain with ample opportunity to prepare for an adulthood where survival depends more on higher cerebral function than on primitive and instinctive qualities of aggression as seen in other animals.

Differential growth patterns The physiological growth of the whole body is but the resultant of the growth of its individual constituent organs and tissues, each having its unique growth characteristics. Growth is not just a uniform process of all organs simply getting larger. Instead, it is made up of a highly complex series of rhythms and different patterns. Suffice it to say that growth of the viscera, brain, lymphoid tissue, fat, reproductive organs and skeleton all follow different patterns, yet surprisingly, with the exception of the brain, only after birth. One aspect of general interest is the growth of tonsils. Between 5 and 10 years of age, their size reaches almost 200% of normal adult size. How many children have been subjected to the machinations of surgeons because of failure to take this physiological occurrence into account!

Changing proportions As part of this mosaic of growth rhythms is the changing proportions of the body found in the growing child. At 18 months, the head is about one quarter of the total length of the body. During the childhood period, the contribution of the head to total body length becomes less, so that at the onset of adolescence it is little over one-eighth the body length. The legs of the young infant constitute about one-third of his body length; at puberty this ratio is nearly one-half due to the relatively greater growth of the lower segment of the body than the trunk. In this passage through childhood the human therefore changes from being short-limbed with a relatively large head to long-limbed with a relatively smaller head.

Tempo of growth The journey towards maturity is achieved at varying rates in different children and which are largely genetically determined: some children move at a moderate tempo, others slowly and some at a presto. The age at which the physical changes of adolescence appear is directly related to this tempo of maturation — the more rapid the rate of maturity, the earlier the onset of puberty. The size of a child at any given age is, however, not a reliable marker of developmental maturity. A child might be small for genetic reasons or because of a slow tempo of maturation.

The measure of developmental maturity (which must not be confused with intellectual maturity) most widely used in clinical practice is that of osseous maturation to determine the *bone age*. To estimate this, an X-ray is taken (usually of the wrist and hand) in order to examine the appearance of various ossification centres (epiphyses) of the wrist, carpus and digits, each of which passes through well-defined visual sequences of development as the bones grow and change their shape. A score is given and from this a measure of bone age ascertained. This description might therefore be a "boy of chronological age of eight years but with a bone age of only six." Boys and girls pass through the same states of skeletal maturity but boys pass more slowly averaging only about 80% the bone age of girls at any one time.

Estimating skeletal maturity is an important clinical tool in the investigation of various growth problems in children, especially short stature, since it will help to determine whether genetic or pathological causes are primarily responsible. It can also be used to help determine ultimate height. The height prediction which can be remarkably accurate (up to 4 cm of final height) has a social application as well as a clinical one: thus in girls wishing to enter ballet school where a uniform height of a *corps de ballet* is desirable, a bone age is often required as a condition for admission in order that an estimate of mature height can be made.

The commonest cause of short stature, itself a common reason for clinical referral to paediatric clinics (see also later), is genetic, not pathological. Children who are more advanced in their physical maturity tend on average to score slightly, but consistently, better in tasks of mental and physical ability than those of the same age and of lesser physical maturity. This might well underlie some of the differences which exist in the school performances of girls and boys. To what extent these differences are due to intrinsic differences in brain maturation or to the social and physical accompaniment of early maturity (confidence, great physical strength, etc.) is not known. No area of developmental biology illustrates more vividly the complex interactions between biological roots and the environment of the child. Under normal circumstances nothing can be done to alter the tempo of development. It is important therefore that those who are responsible for teaching children are aware of the influence on school abilities of differing levels of maturity and where appropriate to make special and sensitive allowances. In many ways it is an anachronism to group children either for educational or athletic pursuits according to chronological age — educationalists please note!

Of the many changes in body composition which take place during childhood, that concerning body fat is amongst the most intriguing. Of the first 3.5 kg of body weight which is synthesized from conception to birth at term, only 11% is fat. The next 3.5 kg gained in the first five months is much higher in fat (40%). The third 3.5 kg synthesized between 5 and 12 months contains much less fat (20%). These changes therefore infer that in the first part of infancy, it is "physiological" to be fat — an important and somewhat paradoxical concept to bear in mind whenever the problem of infant obesity is being considered. The significance of this "physiological fatness" is uncertain although I wonder if it might be Nature's insurance against the precarious period of weaning during which, in unsophisticated conditions, the infant is exceedingly vulnerable to gastrointestinal and other infections which contribute a considerable drain on the body's nutritional economy. I believe that as with other animal species, a plump baby is, providing it is appropriately fed, a healthy baby. There is little to justify the hysteria which continues to be expressed over fat babies. There is no evidence at all that because babies are fat that they will inevitably become fat adults. We would be a far kinder society if we were to care more for the millions of underfed babies than worry about the non-proven consequences of physiological fatness which at its worst simply reflects a parental overindulgence!

Adolescence

Our growth journey reaches its climax at adolescence, an all-embracing term which describes the morphological, physiological and psychological changes which take place in the period of life which links childhood and adulthood and when reproductive capacity is attained. It is a period of great inner and outer change and conflict. Adolescence constitutes three harmoniously interrelated processes which last from about two to five years.

1. *A rapid increase in body size*, established by means of a growth spurt which eventually ends with closure of the epiphyses when adult height is finally reached.
2. *Profound physiological changes in the endocrine system*, especially those which involve the hypothalamopituitary-gonadal axis, leading ultimately to the development of secondary sexual characteristics and the ability to reproduce.
3. *Psychological changes*, many of which are held responsible for what is sometimes termed the "terrible teenage syndrome."

There is considerable variation in the age at which the adolescent growth spurt begins. There are also marked sex differences. Girls on average begin their growth spurt at around ten years of age, about two years sooner than boys. In both sexes the mean duration of the spurt is about three years. The peak growth velocity is greater in boys than in girls but is reached later, about 14 years for boys and 12 years for girls.

The longer preadolescent period of growth, the higher peak velocity and greater gain in height during the spurt accounts for the greater ultimate stature of adult men over women of about 13 cm. Growth in height eventually ceases when the epiphyses close, usually before the age of 18 in boys,

16 in girls. There is, however, a 2% or so further increase in growth into the mid-twenties through continued vertebral column growth. The explanation for the slowing down and eventual cessation of activity of the cartilaginous growth plate remains to be established. It is undoubtedly genetically determined and mediated somehow through a complex endocrine milieu in which growth hormone, androgens and sex hormones all play important roles.

Discord

So much for the harmony of our journey. I would now like to turn to some of its discordant elements. These can be considered in two principal categories. The first is as though the journey has been planned incorrectly from the outset — primary growth disturbances. The second is where the traveller has set out on the normal planned course but the journey has then been distorted from hostile outside forces — *secondary growth disturbances*.

From the outset it is important to be quite clear about one issue. Growth failure is not synonymous with smallness just as growth excess is not synonymous with bigness. A child can be small yet be growing normally just as another child might be of "normal size" yet be failing to grow. Extremes of size are simply *pointers* to possible growth disturbances. This principle, fundamental to the practice of paediatrics, is all too often sadly forgotten and abused. It is responsible for a considerable over-exaggeration of growth problems and undue anxiety on the part of parents. The Victorian poet, J. K. Bangs, anticipated the problem and provides much of the answer!

I met a little Elfman once,
Down where the lilies blow.
I asked him why he was so small and why he did not grow.
He slightly frowned and with his eyes
He looked me through and through.
"I'm quite as big for me," he said
"As you are big for you."

In the following section, I will give some examples of these pathological disturbances to growth. In no way do these reflect prevalence or importance. They simply provide, I hope, interesting examples to illustrate my thesis.

Primary Anomalies of Growth

In these disorders, the fault is in the genetic make-up of the cells of growing organs and tissues, particularly of the skeleton.

The growth of any organism is particularly sensitive to the total amount of its genetic material. The best example of how chromosome abnormalities affect growth is in girls with Turner's Syndrome, who are lacking one of two sex chromosomes. The slower-than-average growth rate, which begins in prenatal life, is progressive through childhood and into adolescence, which does not contain any growth spurt and no other secondary sexual changes, because of absence of the ovaries. The ultimate average height attained in these girls is about 140 cm.

Sometimes inclusion into the genome of one or two abnormal mutant genes can result in serious defects in bone and cartilage growth, many being incompatible with life after birth. In these disorders, there is usually dys-hormonic growth with asymmetry and disproportion in various skeletal dimensions. The brain is often spared. In some there is a well-defined hereditary pattern. *Achondroplasia* (associated throughout the ages with circus clowns), due to mutation of a single gene, is an excellent example of a severe disturbance of growth due to a mutant single gene of large effect.

However diverse their aetiology and presentation, disorders in which the growth failure is due to a primary defect in cell function have two chief features in common. First, growth deficiency begins in the prenatal period. Secondly, there is no effective therapy to recover the deficit of growth rate since the genetic machinery controlling growth is imbalanced from the outset. The growth failure is progressive, the child's height falling steadily farther from the normal during childhood.

Growth excess from primary causes is very rare. I will not dwell on these here.

Secondary Growth Disturbances

In these growth disorders, *growth potential* is normal but is not allowed its optimum expression because of adverse environmental influences originating outside growing cells, obstacles and hazards to the journey. These can (1) deprive growing cells of, or provide them in excess with, substances which are essential for growth (food, hormones and oxygen); (2) interfere with cell function by providing an abnormal extra cellular milieu (as for example in kidney failure); or (3) damage growing cells (as with toxins and infectious agents).

One property common to most of these secondary growth disturbing conditions is that when the cause of growth deficiency is recognized and remedied, "catch-up" phenomenon should occur — *providing the period of growth restriction has not been too long*. I would like to give you some examples of these causes of secondary growth abnormalities.

Growth Failure

Undernutrition

This is the commonest environmental hazard to cause discordant growth. In prenatal life, lack of nutrients may be caused by disease in the mother (such as hypertension) or severe lack of food. When born, these infants are not only underweight for their length (which is also often retarded) but their brains also sometimes show growth constraint. They are likely to suffer the consequences of a low blood sugar during the neonatal period, attributable to low reserves of liver glycogen, unless they are adequately fed. If the period of prenatal growth is a long one, there might also be a permanent deficit in body size attained and even some disturbances in mental functioning, due possibly to interference with brain growth at a critical stage. It is not sufficiently well recognized that prenatal malnutrition is undoubtedly the commonest type of undernutrition seen in children in the developed world.

In postnatal life, lack of food after birth can have an appalling effect on growth, a particularly relevant fact to the two-thirds of the world's children who suffer severe and prolonged protein and calorie malnutrition. An estimate is that about twelve million children each year will die from this deprivation. As I mentioned earlier, even more will suffer the long-term consequences of malnutrition. This appalling scourge usually begins after weaning when there is too little food available and that which is available is of poor nutritional value and likely to be contaminated.

In developed parts of the world, a primary lack of food after birth is unusual. The most common cause is probably early lactation failure, which can slow down the growth of the whole body.

Impaired Digestion and Absorption of Food

Several syndromes of malabsorption result in a failure of nutrients to reach growing tissues — a type of secondary undernutrition. Of these, coeliac disease, an abnormal reaction of the gut to the wheat protein gluten, and cystic fibrosis (in which as part of widespread exocrine gland malfunctions, there is malabsorption of fat due to pancreatic insufficiency), which are well recognized in European children, are surprisingly absent in the Chinese.

Endocrine Disturbances

As I mentioned, hormones play an important role in influencing cell growth. There are two principal disorders of the endocrine glands which can adversely affect growth.

The first is *growth hormone deficiency*. This, though exceedingly rare — 1/40,000 births in European populations — has provided a vital model to understand much of the physiology of normal growth. Children who lack growth hormone will end up as adults only about 130 cm tall. They fall into two categories. Firstly, those in whom there is idiopathic (cause unknown) growth hormone deficiency, either isolated or associated with other anterior pituitary hormone deficiencies (hypopituitarism). In these children, there is no obvious growth deficit in prenatal life. It is most commonly diagnosed at about the age of 5 or 6; when children start school, they are noted by their parents to be extremely small compared with their friends. In their external features, children with idiopathic growth hormone deficiency appear doll-like with an increase in subcutaneous fat and normal skeletal proportions. Intellectually they arc normal. Thc sccond group of children in whom growth hormone deficiency can develop is where the hypothalamus/anterior pituitary gland has been destroyed by other malignant infiltration's or cranial irradiation in the course of treating leukaemia.

The second important endocrine disorder to interfere with growth is that of *thyroid hormone deficiency*. In view of the fundamental role of thyroid hormones in brain growth and protein synthesis in the skeleton, it is not surprising that deficiencies of thyroid hormones will cause growth failure in both fetal and postnatal life as well as severe mental impairment. The origin of this thyroid abnormality is either abnormal descent of the thyroid gland or metabolic errors in the synthesis of thyroid hormones or in older children destruction of a previously normal thyroid gland by circulating antibodies. In these older children, there is growth failure associated with delayed bone maturation and abnormal appearance of the epiphyses. With treatment, providing the disorder is diagnosed soon after birth, there is complete "catch-up" and no residual mental disorder.

Psycho-social Growth Failure

Not all these obstacles to normal growth are "organic." *Psycho-social growth failure* is well recognized to be associated with stunting of growth. Usually these children are aged between 3 and 8 (although no age is beyond all risk), living in very poor social conditions and emotionally deprived. In many instances, there is global retardation in growth with infantile proportions of the skeleton (short legs in relation to the rest of the body) retained. These features presumably reflect the chronicity of the growth-retarding influences. In young infants, the principal growth disturbance is that of failure to thrive — poor weight gain associated with wasting of subcutaneous fat. Reasons for psycho-social growth failure are complex. They include poor food intake from a blunted appetite together with an overall depression of endocrine function related to depressed growth hormone levels. Indeed, the features are more typical of an adaptation to malnutrition than an adaptation to primary endocrine disease. Behavioural disturbances are invariably present in these children including an air of submissive apathy, much of which might even be seen as an adaptation to conserve all available energy.

Miscellaneous Causes

Other hazards to cause growth retardation are lack of oxygen as found in children with severe cyanotic heart disease and chronic lung disease and the accumulation of toxic products of metabolism in children with renal failure. In this latter group, growth failure is likely to be related to failure to excrete organic acids and other waste substances which accumulate in the extra-cellular milieu, thereby "poisoning" growth processes.

Toxins, Drugs and Infectious Agents — Environmental Hazards

Finally I would like to mention briefly growth failure due to harmful environmental influences. Infectious agents (such as rubella virus) and drugs (for example, thalidomide) mostly have their disruptive effects on growth potential primarily in the embryonic and early fetal periods. Growth disturbance in this period can cause multiple errors of morphogenesis and at the same time interfere with mechanisms which control growth. Depending on the nature and the timing of the insult will be the type of growth disturbance. For example, rubella contracted during the embryonic period will cause a plethora of distorted organ growth (heart defects, brain anomalies, cataracts, deafness, etc.) as well as retarding total body growth. Infection after the embryonic period will leave relatively unscathed organ growth yet physical size will be affected.

It is now recognized that one of the most important toxins which can interfere with growth in prenatal life is alcohol. Excessive consumption of alcohol taken in the first half of pregnancy will result in infants born with several dysmorphic facial features, occasional defects in the heart and limbs and overall growth retardation. Considerable interest is currently being given to this problem.

Growth Excess

Problems of growth excess (macrosomia) are few. I wish to mention only one condition — namely, the baby born to a poorly controlled diabetic mother who is allowing too much sugar to cross the placenta, thereby stimulating fetal insulin release and causing excess laying down of sugar as fat and also probably enhancing skeletal growth. The better controlled the maternal diabetes, the less the chances of macrosomia.

Conclusion

So much for our journey. I hope I have given some insight into one of the great fascinations of human biology, namely the growth of the child. Without a thorough understanding of these growth processes, there can be no real understanding of paediatrics. Medical students in general are launched too soon into the diseases of children before having found time to assimilate the normal patterns of growth. It is for this reason that in this Faculty, along with many others in the world, a course of normal growth and development is now very much a part of the course in basic sciences. After all, growth itself is but an amalgam of all the basic sciences.

The study of growth in Hong Kong children, both in health and in disease, will be a major part of our departmental research programme.

Already we have been fortunate to receive generous support from the Croucher Foundation in Hong Kong to investigate a local anxiety that growth failure from poor feeding practices might still be a problem here. Twenty years ago Dr. Flora Baber, with Professor Elaine Field, had the foresight to undertake a prospective study of the growth in a large number of Hong Kong children. They produced what can only be described as a true classic in paediatric literature for this part of the world — *Growing Up in Hong Kong*. We intend to build on this foundation and follow in their footsteps, difficult though this will be. Maybe "Growing Up in Sha Tin" will be the result! Detailed studies of growth patterns in children with heart disease, those born prematurely and of extreme size at birth will also be undertaken, to name but a few other examples of intended research.

I hope that members of our young Department, by working harmoniously both together and with many others who care for children in home, hospital and community, will make a contribution to allow our children travel their journey of growth and development as harmoniously as possible, and when discord strikes, to give them and their families the sympathy, care, love and attention they need to minimize their burden.

2

Genetic Influences on Growth in Length with Particular Reference to Children of Asiatic Origin

The Hong Kong Journal of Paediatrics, 1986; 3:193–203

Summary

Genetic factors undoubtedly account for differences in size between individuals within any ethnic group. More contentious is the extent to which genetic factors account for variations in the size of children of major racial groups. Early growth characteristics of Asiatic (Chinese, Japanese and Indo-Malayan) children studied over the past couple of decades differ from those of other major racial groups, showing a faltering over the first couple of years of postnatal life. It is argued that this feature is likely to be more of genetic than environmental origin, making a major contribution to smaller adult stature. These findings, which need further substantiation from studies in children born at the present time, have important implications not only for the management of individual clinical problems but also in the epidemiological definition of growth failure in childhood populations.

Introduction

Just as the growth curve of any child from conception through to the adolescent climax is the outward expression of an interaction between its genetic potential and environment, so also will the growth curve of populations reflect this interaction. Growth of long bones and vertebrae on which body stature depends takes place under the influence of intermediary growth factors through activities within the growth plate, a zone of dividing cartliage cells separating the primary from secondary ossification centre and which deposit substances containing mineral salts to form the bone matrix. As the rate of growth slows, so does the growth plate become narrower until eventually bone in the main shaft joins with bone in the epiphysis, eliminating the growth plate in the process. No further growth is then possible, the epiphysis being "closed." At the same time as bone growth takes place, constant remodelling and moulding also occur in order to sustain the changes in shape demanded by the growing skeleton. For normal skeletal growth to take place, dividing cells must be provided with an optimum metabolic milieu supplying energy, amino acids, vitamins, fatty acids, minerals and various endocrine secretions. Without balanced provision of these substances, growth will fail and a genetically endowed physical growth potential will not be realized.

Faltering of linear growth rate — the process of stunting — is one of the most sensitive of all measures of socio-economic adversity both in individuals and populations, surpassing infant mortality since it is concerned with the nutritional and health experiences of the living. The matter is however not quite so straightforward since the appearance of faltering on growth charts (downward centile crossing) can sometimes be physiological and under genetic influence. An understanding of genetic influences on growth is therefore essential for the correct interpretation of patterns of growth both at an individual and population level. It is this issue to which this chapter addresses itself.

"One of Man's Most Heritable Traits"

In 1989, Francis Galton in his treatise *Natural Inheritance* recognized the "beautiful regularity" in the stature of a population that shows "small dependence on differences of bringing up."[1] Along with recognition of height with mid-parental size in individual children, he was among the first to scientifically document stature as "one of man's most heritable traits" and in so doing began the quest for better understanding of genetic influences on the control of growth. The impact of polygenic influences on skeletal growth is evident in many ways — variations of size between individuals within the same ethnic group; higher coefficiency for height between monozygotic than dizygotic twins; the close relationship between the mean height of parents and mature stature of their offspring and the differences between the growth curves of boys and girls with the earlier puberty growth spurt in girls and in boys a higher peak growth velocity — to give but a few examples.[2] Where there is abnormal genetic make-up, stature is often affected, as for example in Turner's Syndrome,[3] Down's Syndrome[4] and many conditions dictated by abnormal single genes, such as achondroplasia. These examples, in both normal and abnormal children, leave no doubt as to the importance of genetic factors in controlling and directing the growth programme, though how in individual children this genetic control, coded in the DNA template, is transcribed into actual processes is still incompletely understood.

Timing of Physiological Genetic Influences

In all living organisms there exists an intrinsic "genetic momentum" which permits a minimum growth performance even under the most hostile of environmental conditions. Of particular fascination is that genetic influences unique to an individual child really come into their own after birth.

Growth in prenatal life is heavily influenced by the mother through the intra-uterine environment she provides for the fetus. At this focal point converge her own genetic make-up, nutrient intake, health (past and present) and lifestyle (in particular cigarette consumption). So dominant are these intra-uterine environmental influences that the fetal genome has been estimated to account for only about 20% of the variance in birth size.[5] This powerful maternal control (its mechanisms as yet poorly identified although it is now becoming increasingly evident that uterine size plays an important role) on fetal growth, totally dominating at this stage of development any paternal influences, was first recognized by Walton and Hammond in their studies in 1938 of Shetland pony/shire crosses.[6] It has probably evolved in order to allow the safest possible conditions for parturition and thereby survival of the species. For this control to function effectively, the fetal genotype must be subservient to local maternal environmental influences, especially those with the capacity to constrain growth. At birth, correlation of length with mid-parental height is only about 0.2 but this changes rapidly over the subsequent 18 months or so when it reaches its adult value of 0.5: correlation of length at birth with adult height is also small (about 0.3) but by the age of 3 it has risen to 0.8.[2] These improvements in height correlations with time are phenotypic expressions of the growth genotype brought into play once the child is freed at birth from prenatal maternal influences. When considered against a background of conventional clinical centile standards these genetically controlled "target seeking and self stabilizing" effects[7] are often seen as growth tracking with trajectories moving in either upward ("catch-up") or downward ("lag down") directions. The best study so far on the subject is from the late Professor David Smith and his colleagues in Seattle.[8] It has shown that in well-nourished, healthy American babies, about two-thirds of children crossed more than one centile line over the first year against a seven-point centile grid (97, 90, 75, 50, 25, 10, 3). Those of extreme size at birth showed greatest tracking* in both upward and downward directions.

The first couple of years after birth is therefore a period when the expression of genes controlling the growth programme emerge out of the shadow of maternal intra-uterine influences in order to direct the individual baby's growth trajectory into its genetically predetermined channel (genetic influences do not have another such major effect until the puberty growth spurt) (Figure 1). It is this that explains the remarkable heterogeneity of growth profiles in individual babies over this time. Interpretation of growth profiles at this developmental stage is therefore sometimes difficult, having to make allowances for the phenomenon of physiological tracking. Whenever a growth shift is found, it is important to bear in mind that genetic influences might be a possible cause, in addition to those of more environmental origin. Failure to do so may sometimes, in the case of downward tracking, give rise to a mistaken diagnosis of growth failure, although this statement will obviously apply less to children in socio-economically poor countries where environmental effects on growth overshadow the more subtle genetic influences than to children brought up in more privileged environments.

Are There Genetic Origins to Differences That Exist in the Stature between Different Races?

It is against this background of genetic variation of stature and growth between individuals that I would now like to turn to a more contentious

---

* The terms "tracking," "shifts," "deviations," "centile crossings" are used synonymously in this chapter to denote movement of growth curves in either upward or downward directions.

Figure 1. The Genetically Predetermined Channel of a Baby Comes into Effect at Birth out of the Shadow of Maternal Intra-uterine Influence.

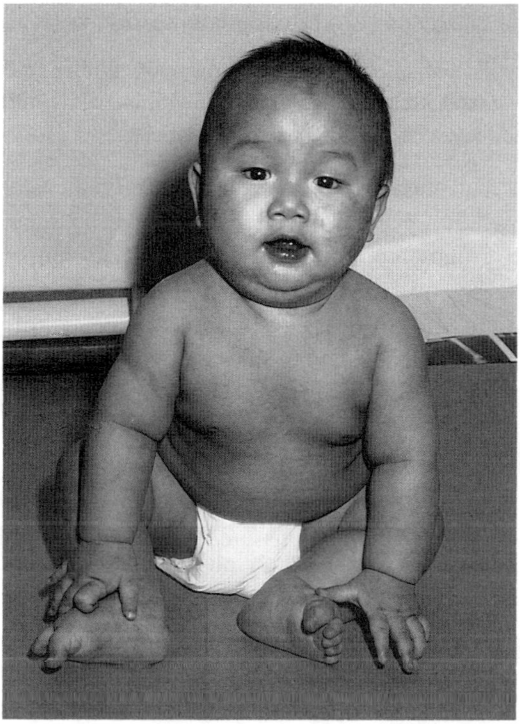

issue and the major thesis of this chapter, namely the extent to which genetic factors account for the diversity in physical size that exists between children of different races.

Examining the physical attributes of the many groups of mankind can not but fail to remind of dramatic genetic influences. Colour of skin, nature and distribution of body hair, body type, physical proportions and body composition, rate of maturation are but a few examples of the remarkable ways in which various human subgroups have, over aeons of time, evolved and preserved, through natural selection, very varied physical characteristics to help them be accommodated in, and allow satisfactory adaptation to, very diverse geographical habitats. The scope of Nature's ability to adapt to widely differing ecological niches cannot be better demonstrated.

It is therefore surprising (at least to me) to discover that where stature of young children is the physical characteristic under debate, this is considered by many authorities to be little affected by ethnic differences. The following statement from a paper by Habicht and colleagues from Guatemala and published in the *Lancet* of 1974 provides an illustration.

> From data collected among privileged groups of children in developing countries, we have concluded that child growth is mainly influenced by social economic status and not by race or ethnicity.[9]

Yet no one can surely doubt the genetic origins of very obvious differences that exist between the adult heights of well-nourished and healthy different racial groups brought up in privileged environments that have allowed genetic potential to achieve its full, uninhibited potential.[10] Are protagonists of the equal or near similar growth potential of various racial groups in early childhood implying that these differences emerge later in childhood?

Whether or not genetic factors are responsible for different patterns of growth between races is central to the continuing controversy of the appropriateness of reference growth standards to judge the adequacy of growth in individuals and populations and therefore ultimately to the definition of growth insufficiency.[11] Those who adhere to the view of equal growth potential during early childhood for children of all races favour the notion that growth standards developed from European populations in industrialized countries are appropriate for all children populations and can therefore be used as a tool to survey epidemiologically the problem of growth failure. Whilst admitting to the obvious that appalling stunting of growth is caused by malnutrition and other environmental scourges, can we disregard gene pools of different racial groups in their differential influences on early growth? I believe not.

To argue my case, I would first like to trace some of the recent history of this contentious issue. One of the key studies to which we are referred is that of Habicht and his colleagues.[9] Writing in the *Lancet* in 1974, they compared growth in height and weight over the first five years in samples of children (presumably) well-nourished from developed countries (the United States, Britain, Australia) with children in developing countries, urban and rural assumed to be considerably undernourished (India, Columbia, Guatemala, Thailand). The overall differences between children's heights from developed countries were small (3%). In contrast, differences between these children and those living in poor urban and rural regions were much higher, approaching 12% and as high as 30% for weight. Differences due to race were therefore small compared with environmental effects.

> We see no way to demonstrate with this kind of data that the small difference in growth found between different ethnic groups are due to genetic factors.

The authors concluded that growth standards derived from well-to-do children in developed countries should serve as an optimum standard of reference for all children.

In 1981, Graitcer and Gentry from Atlanta, Georgia, analysed heights and weights of 2,366 children aged 6 months to 5 years from privileged areas of Haiti, Egypt and Togo (private day care centres, paediatricians offices and families of government and military officials), populations representing principally peoples of African and Indo-Mediterranean origin.[12] These were compared with the reference standards from the National Centre for Health Statistics (NCHS) (derived from healthy, non-institutionalized American children), the growth standard now widely used and recommended as a reference curve to judge the adequacy of growth in childhood.[13] (It is not sufficiently well appreciated that these standards are based on quite old data. For children under the age of 3, which is particularly relevant to the topic under discussion in this chapter, the measurements were collected between 1929 and 1975.) The authors found that the 5th, 50th and 95th centiles were very close to the reference population and concluded, as had Habicht,[9] that

> when adverse environmental influences such as increased exposure to infection and decreased food intake are optimized, ethnic and geographical differences have little if any influence on growth.

They likewise recommended the use of one reference for all countries to evaluate the impact of environmental hostile factors on the growth of pre-school children. Professor John Waterlow in a letter to the *Lancet* in 1980 wrote:

> I am inclined to think that growth potential in the early years of life is not much affected by ethnic differences. If that is so it seems justifiable to apply North American, European standards internationally.[14]

A leading article in the *Lancet* in 1984 authoritatively seemed to put the lid on the argument with the statement that

> the controversy of whether or not growth standards for children developed in Europe and North America are universally applicable appears now to be settled in favour of those who maintain that they are.[11]

It reinforced the notion that the growth of privileged groups of children in developing countries does not differ importantly from these standards. But this brings us to the kernel of the problem: What is important? I believe any difference to be important, however small, if it has such an effect on professional opinion so as to influence and change dietary practices and other aspects of health care.

What impresses me however is that in the studies referred to, and which have considerable influence on recent thinking concerning genetic influences on early growth, little reference has been made to children of Asiatic origin — Chinese, Japanese and Indo-Malays — who make up more than a quarter of mankind. Several studies have shown that Asiatic children at maturity are smaller than those of other ethnic groups. For example in 1965, Ashcroft in Jamaica studied the size of 5,000 children aged 11–17 years, attending eight fee-paying secondary schools in Kingston from upper and middle socio-economic classes status.[15] The statures of African, Afro-European and European children were similar, indicating a similar potential for growth in height: that of the Chinese children was however consistently smaller. Thus, at 11 years the boys were 3 cm shorter. An earlier puberty growth spurt saw this narrow to about 2 cm at 13 years but the gap then widened until at 17 years, the differences between the Chinese children and those of African and European origin amounted to about 7 cm. Ashcroft was firmly of the opinion that this difference was genetic in origin. Barr and his colleagues from San Francisco in 1972 also showed in 7,500 children aged 5 to 14 years that in general children of "yellow skin" were markedly shorter and lighter than white and black children.[16] I therefore contend that before the case for a similar early genetic growth potential can be accepted for all races, the early growth of Asiatic children must be analysed in further detail and compared with that of other populations.

Linear Growth in Asiatic Children

A recent paper[17] has described the growth during the first two years of life of Hong Kong children studied in the 1960s[18] and late 1970s[19] compared with NCHS standards[13] and concluded that marked downward tracking occurs between 6–18 months. An argument was put forward that a large part of this trend could well be physiological and not necessarily the consequence of inadequate nutrition during the weaning period. I have now extended the analysis to include other populations of Asiatic children — eight sets of growth data published over the past twenty years or so from Japan,[20,21] Singapore,[22] Korea,[23] Thailand,[24] Taiwan.[25] Children contributing to these studies were brought up in what were then generally considered by the various authors to be favourable socio-economic conditions. Indeed, many of the data provide normal reference standards for clinical use. An overall growth curve has been constructed from the mean heights at various ages over the first five years (1, 3, 6, 9, 12 months, and 2, 3, 4, 5 years) and compared with the NCHS curves, in view of the recommendations for the ubiquitous adoption of these reference standards. I accept from the outset that there are several sources of error and inconsistency in my approach to these intra-ethnic comparisons — differences in sizes of population studied, different methods of measurement, diversities in environmental conditions, variable time of assessment, to give but a few. Admitting to these, I do believe that the resulting mean growth curve closely approximates to the truth about what is currently known about the physical growth of Asiatic children.

Over the first year, the average percentage difference in height measured at five points (1, 3, 6, 9 and 12 months) between the biggest and smallest Asiatic populations was about 3%, and from 1–5 years, about 4%. Figure 2 shows the mean growth curves against the NCHS data. During the first few months or so, growth in length follows a remarkably similar pattern. Thereafter there begins a very definite period of downward tracking which continues for a few years before levelling off.

A more quantifiable and universally preferred method for presenting anthropometric data can be obtained by analysing changes in the Standard Deviation Score (Z score) of the NCHS standards (Figure 3). In both boys and girls there is, over the first three years, a downward shift of approximately two standard deviations. Over the next two years, there is an impression of some upward shift but not to any meaningful extent.

Figure 2. Mean Curves of Growth in Length from Birth to 5 Years in Asiatic Boys and Girls[18–25] Compared with the NCHS Reference Standards.[13]

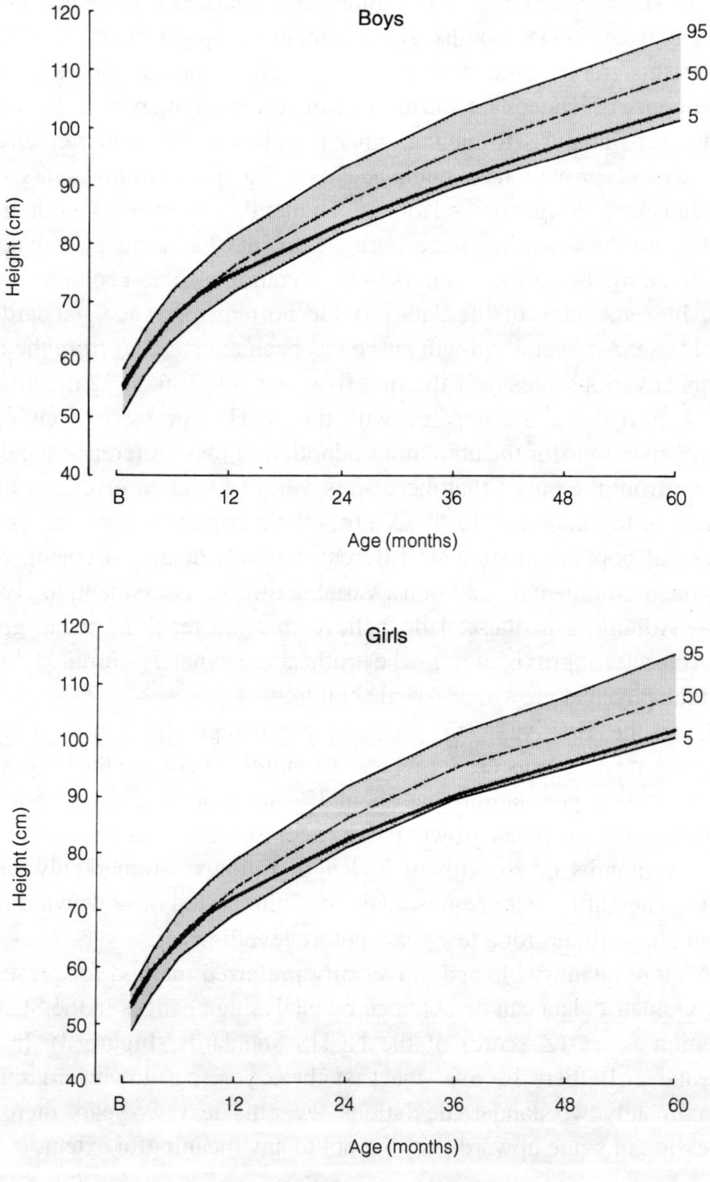

Figure 3. Changes in the Mean S.D.S. Score of Asiatic Children[18–25] in Relation to the NCHS Standards.

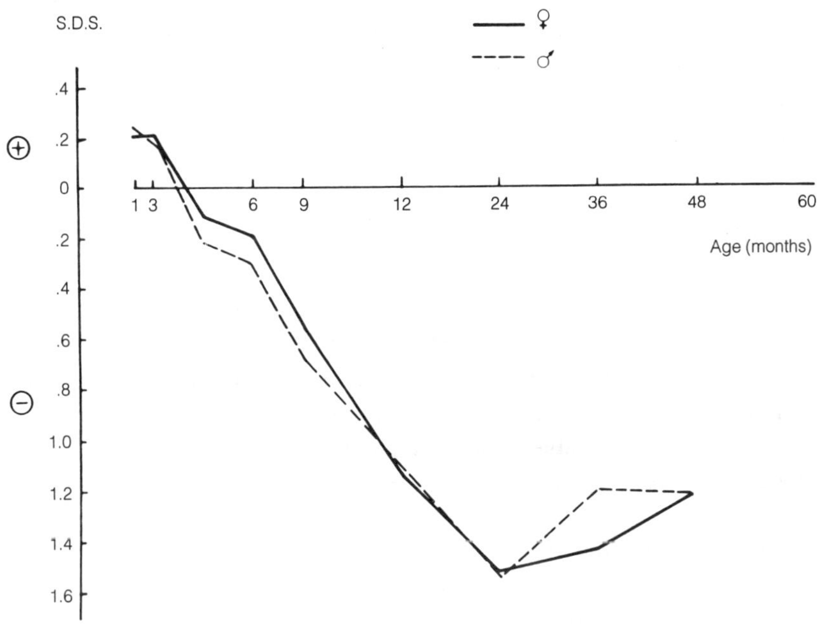

As previously mentioned, the data in several of the studies referred to are being widely used in their various countries as reference growth standards. It is not recorded that the children were anything other than healthy, although it is possible that within the group as a whole, some children's growth might have faltered for pathological reasons. It is difficult therefore to avoid concluding that the character of early growth of Asiatic children during the first few years after birth is different from that of the NCHS standard — and by inference also from that of Black children who, if brought up in a favourable environment, will have a growth potential similar to that of European children.[10] If the early period of growth faltering was principally due to environmental influences, for example undernutrition over the weaning period, "catch-up" would have been expected after this time with provision of a good, well-balanced diet. This seems not to take place. This hypothesis might be challenged on the grounds that some data used are dated, therefore not accurately reflecting secular changes that have taken place over the past couple of decades.[26] To meet this criticism, in Figure 4 are described mean growth curves of babies measured within the past ten years in Hong Kong (1978)[19] and Taiwan (1984)[27] (the latter having only recently been drawn to my attention). Both studies are of healthy children. The overall growth profiles are similar to that of the larger group supporting the contention that the growth curve in Asiatic children is distinctive, but more for physiological than environmental reasons. Why this should be so is outside the brief of this chapter.

Conclusion

My interpretation of the relevance of genetic factors to growth in length in early childhood can be summarized as follows.

First, differences in genetic make-up undoubtedly account for variations in size between individuals within any ethnic group and who are brought up in comparable environmental conditions. This genotype has a particularly strong effect in the first few years after birth when the child moves away from heavy maternal influences on prenatal growth. This often results in considerable shifts in both upward as well as downward directions which must be always borne in mind whenever making a judgement on the profile of early growth in an individual child. These shifts are greater in children born at the extremes of size.

Second, variations in size between different racial groups, even allowing for hostile environmental factors, can also have a genetic basis. Pronouncements on a uniformity of genetic growth potential in infants and young children of the major racial groups do not apply when children of Asiatic origin are compared with those of European and African origin. The early growth characteristics of Asiatic children differ in their basic profile in showing a deceleration of growth rate over the first couple of years of postnatal life. Viewed on the NCHS growth curves, these are shown as downward tracking from the first through to the third years of life and a continuation thereafter in lower centile channels. These characteristics of the Asiatic growth curve are likely to be more of genetic than environmental origin and make a major contribution to later overall smaller adult stature.

Third, the magnitude of these differences of genetic origin do not approach those that can be caused through malnutrition and other sources

Figure 4. Mean Curves of Growth in Length in Recently Studied Hong Kong[19] (----) and Taiwan[27] (—) Boys and Girls Compared with the NCHS Reference Standards.[13]

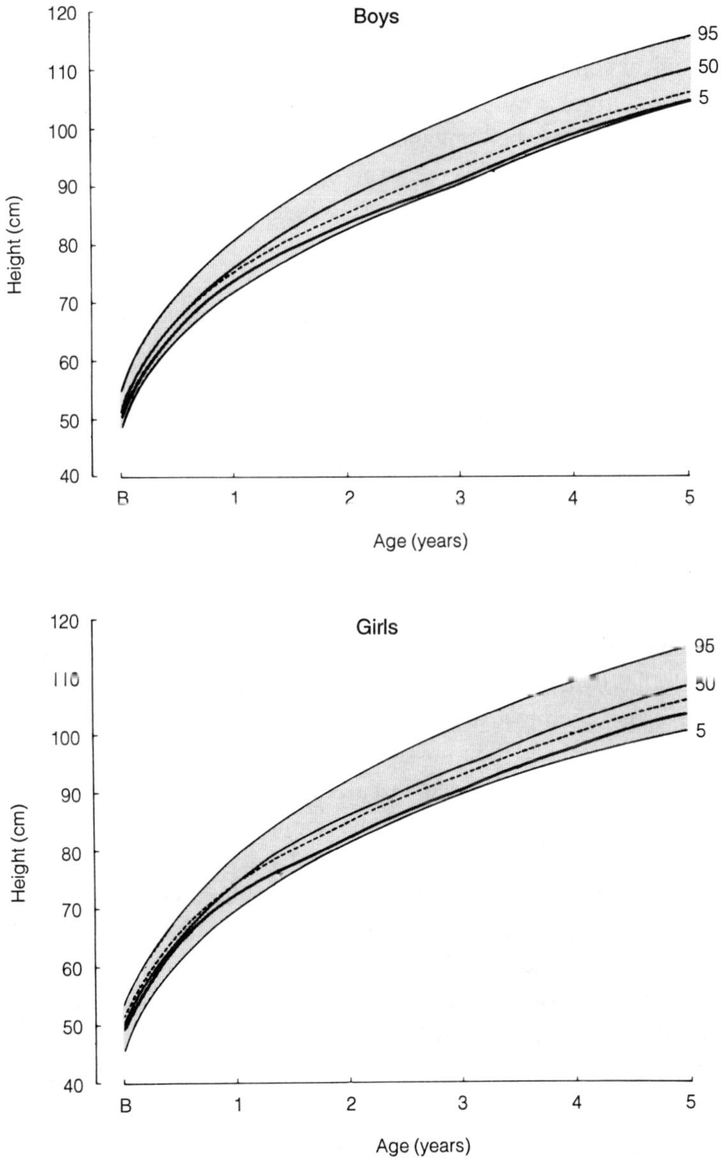

of environmental deprivation where 10–20% differences from the NCHS median are commonly described with downward shifts of up to three standard deviations over the first few years. But I do not believe they should be disregarded. They can for example be sufficient to query the validity of using the NCHS reference standard for Asiatic children to assess on a population basis, growth faltering. Furthermore, failure to recognize a sizeable physiological contribution to the period of early lag-down growth can lead to mistaken attitudes by professional people to such an extent that wrong feeding practices may be implemented in an attempt to reverse the trend.

There is a danger of this occurring in Hong Kong where (prematurely I believe) the interpretation of faltering as being due to nutritional deficiencies has given rise to unnecessary concern. In August 1983, the front page of the *South China Morning Post* led with the following headline — "HK Babies Go Hungry, Say Studies." The newspaper article drew attention to the fact that "about one fifth of Hong Kong babies are severely undernourished in the crucial period between the ages of seven months and two years." Another statement was particularly emotive and disconcerting:

> If we are justified in assuming that head size reflects brain mass it may be that the undernutrition of these infants was sufficient to interrupt the period of active brain growth resulting in diminished potential for future performance.

In the study referred to, blame was given to a bad weaning diet of calorie and vitamin deficient congee (soft watery rice) during weaning. Recent studies by Dr. Anita Li and her colleagues in the University of Hong Kong have also continued to draw attention to supposedly poor diets during the weaning period and their possible impact on early growth.[28]

Further studies are needed to carefully examine growth patterns of Chinese and other children of Asiatic origin in relation to their nutrient intake. Especially important is to critically evaluate the relevance of recommended dietary allowances (RDA) to children who might well have different physiological growth characteristics from those on whom RDA were originally obtained. Particular attention must be given to children born now in view of obvious secular changes that have taken place over the past few decades together with profound changes in feeding practices. Even leaving aside the issue of the desirability or otherwise of an internationally accepted growth standard as an epidemiological tool for quantifying malnutrition in different countries, it is essential that we have reliable growth standards for the routine day-to-day clinical use in individual children for the reliable assessment of their clinical problems.

Acknowledgements

I thank Miss Angela Yan for her time and patience in typing this manuscript.

References

1. Galton, F. *Natural Inheritance*. London: McMillan and Company, 1889.
2. Tanner, J. M. Physical Growth and Development. In Forfar, J. O., and Arneil, G. C., eds., *Textbook of Paediatrics*, Vol. 1, 3rd Ed. London: Churchill Livingstone, 1984.
3. Lyon, A. J., Preece, M. A., and Grant, D. B. Growth Curve for Girls with Turner Syndrome. *Arch Dis Child*, 1985; 60:932–35.
4. Cronk, C. E. Growth of Children with Down's Syndome: Birth to Age 3 Years. *Pediatrics*, 1978; 61:564–68.
5. Polani, P. E. Chromosomal and Other Genetic Influence on Birth Weight Variation. In *Size at Birth*. Ciba Symposium 27 (new series). Amsterdam: Associated Scientific Publishers, 1974; 127–59.
6. Walton, A., and Hammond, J. The Maternal Effects on Growth and Conformation in Shire Horse–Shetland Pony Crosses. *Proc R Soc Biol*, 1938; 125: 311–24.
7. Tanner, J. M. Regulation of Growth in Size of Mammals. *Nature*, 1963; 199:845–47.
8. Smith, D. W., Truog, W., Rogers, J. E., *et al.* Shifting Linear Growth during Infancy and the Genetics of Growth in Fetal Life through Infancy. *J Pediatr*, 1976; 89:225–34.
9. Habicht, J. P., Martorell, R., Yarbrough, C., *et al.* Height and Weight Standards for Pre-school Children. How Relevant Are Ethnic Differences in Growth Potential? *Lancet*, 1974; 1:611–15.
10. Eveleth, P. B., and Tanner, J. M. *Worldwide Variation in Human Growth*. IBP Synthesis Series 8. Cambridge: Cambridge University Press, 1976.
11. A Measure of Agreement on Growth Standards (editorial). *Lancet*, 1984; 1:142–43.
12. Graitcer, P. H., and Gentry, E. M. Measuring Children: One Reference for All. *Lancet*, 1981; 2:297–99.
13. Hammill, P.V.V., Drizd, T. A., Johnson, C. L., Reid, R. B., Rouche, A. F., and Moore, W. M. Physical Growth: National Centre for Health Statistics Centiles. *Am J Clin Nutr*, 1979; 32:607–96.

14. Waterlow, J. C. Child Growth Standrads (letter). *Lancet*, 1980; 1:717.
15. Ashcroft, M. T., Heneage, P., and Lovell, H. G. Heights and Weights of Jamaican School Children of Various Ethnic Groups. *Am J Phys Anthrop*, 1964; 24:35–44.
16. Barr, G. D., Allen, C. M., and Shinefield, H. R. Height and Weight of 7,500 Children of 3 Skin Colours. Pediatric Multiphasic Program: Report No. 3. *Am J Dis Child*, 1972; 124:866–72.
17. Davies, D. P., and Leung, S. F. Growth of Hong Kong Infants during the First Two Years of Life. *Early Hum Dev*, 1985; 11:247–54.
18. Chang, K.S.F., Lee, M. M., Low, W. D., *et al.* Standards of Height and Weight of Southern Chinese Children. *Far East Med J*, 1965; 1:101–9.
19. Survey on Weight, Height and Head Circumference of Pre-school Children in April 1978. Family Health Service and Statistical Unit, Medical and Health Department. *Hong Kong Soc Community Med HK Bull*, 1980; 45–57.
20. Tokyo Department of Maternal and Child Health. Physical Status of Japanese Children in 1970. Department of Maternal and Child Health Institute of Public Health, Tokyo.
21. Terada, H., and Hoshi, H. Longitudinal Study on the Physical Growth in Japanese, Growth in Lengths of Extremities during the First Three Years of Life. *Acta Anatomica Nipponica*, 1965; 41:313–26.
22. Wong, H. B., Tye, C. Y., and Quek, K. M. Anthropometric Studies on Singapore Children: Heights, Weights and Skull Circumference on Pre-school Children. *J Singapore Paediatr Soc*, 1972; 14:68–69.
23. Korea Ministry of Health. Growth Data of Korean Children. *J Korean Pediatr Assoc*, 1967; 10 (Supplement No. 4).
24. Khanjanasthiti, P., Supchaturas, P., Mekanandha, P., *et al.* The Anthropometry of the Growth of Infant and Pre-school Children (unpublished manuscript). Cited in Eveleth and Tanner (Reference 10).
25. Shih, S. C., Wu, T. H., and Chen, K. P. Growth Charts of Height and Chest and Head Circumference for Children under 6 Years of Age in Taiwan. *J Form Med Assoc*, 1966; 65:313–25.
26. Fung, K. P., Lau, S. P., Chow, O.K.W., *et al.* A Survey on Growth of Hong Kong Children. *HK J Paediatr*, 1985; 2:105–16.
27. Lu, C. C., Wu, T. C., Wu, J. R., *et al.* Studies on Body Height, Weight, Head Gain and Chest Girth on Normal Healthy Children in Kaohsiung City. *Acta Paediatr Sin*, 1980; 21:17–25.
28. Li, A.M.C., Baber, F. M., Yu, A.M.C., *et al.* The Weaning Diet of Hong Kong Children. *Journal HKMA*, 1985; 37:167–75.

3

*Nutritional Problems in Infancy and Early Childhood: A Commentary on the Contemporary Hong Kong Scene**

The Hong Kong Journal of Paediatrics, 1988; 5 (Suppl.):135–51

Summary

The view is put forward, supported by some recently collected data from a large sample of young infants being followed up in Sha Tin (New Territories) for their growth, well-being and nutritional status, that there now unlikely exists any significant undernutrition in Hong Kong children during pre-weaning and weaning periods. Specific examples offered include adequacy of iron and calcium intakes, normal vitamin D levels in plasma, satisfactory energy, and more than ample protein intake. Growth patterns show deviation from the National Centre for Health Statistics (NCHS) reference curves after about 6 months but this, it is argued, is more likely to be a normal physiological profile. Such greatly improved nutrient status during weaning that has taken place over the past 25 years is the result of milk formula being continued well into the second year and a wide range of weaning foods (meat, vegetable, rice, fruit) being given from 6 months onwards along with congee (soft watery rice). Major credit for such improvements must go to the maternal and child health (MCH) clinics where most education on infant nutrition is given to mothers.

---

* Based on a paper presented at an International Workshop on "Early Childhood Nutritional Problems in the Far East" organized jointly by the Department of Paediatrics, The Chinese University of Hong Kong, and the Hong Kong Paediatric Society in November 1987.

These findings in Sha Tin contrast with studies in the early 1980s from two other parts of Hong Kong, Kwun Tong and Aberdeen, when concern was expressed over the nutritional adequacy of the weaning diet. Arguments are put forward which include that these latter observations might have been unduly pessimistic. The further study of growth and nutrition in other parts of Hong Kong is nevertheless urged in order to provide as comprehensive a picture as possible of contemporary nutrient status in infancy and early childhood in order to judge the overall applicability of our findings.

Introduction

Nutrient intake in infancy and early childhood performs many functions:

1. to provide building blocks and energy for optimum physical growth and its accompanying physiological changes;
2. to satisfy the need of normal body functions for essential metabolic substances;
3. to help protect from infectious diseases, especially gastroenteritis and perhaps antigen-provoked disorders (such as eczema and asthma) and respiratory infections.
4. to sow the seeds of an attitude for a good diet in later life and maybe to programme later metabolic events so as to lessen the risks of diet-related disorders, particularly cardiovascular disease.

These requirements can be met by providing in the diet of the young child a balance of energy, protein, fat, carbohydrate, vitamins and minerals (and, for the breast-fed baby immunoglobulins and other protective substances). When these needs are satisfied, we can then propose that optimum nutrition has been achieved. How near are we in Hong Kong to meeting this nutritional ideal? In this chapter, I will be exploring this question, examining our infants' diet and its major consequences for physical growth and some nutrient-related disorders.

For the benefit of colleagues from overseas can I offer a backdrop for this presentation. Hong Kong compromises Hong Kong Island, Kowloon Peninsular and New Territories which itself is made up of mainland and over 200 islands of various sizes. The total area is about 460 square miles and made up of large urban conurbations interspersed with rural areas much

Figure 1. Sha Tin New Town. An Example of a Planned New Town in the Hong Kong New Territories in Order to Provide Accommodation for a Progressively Expanding Population.

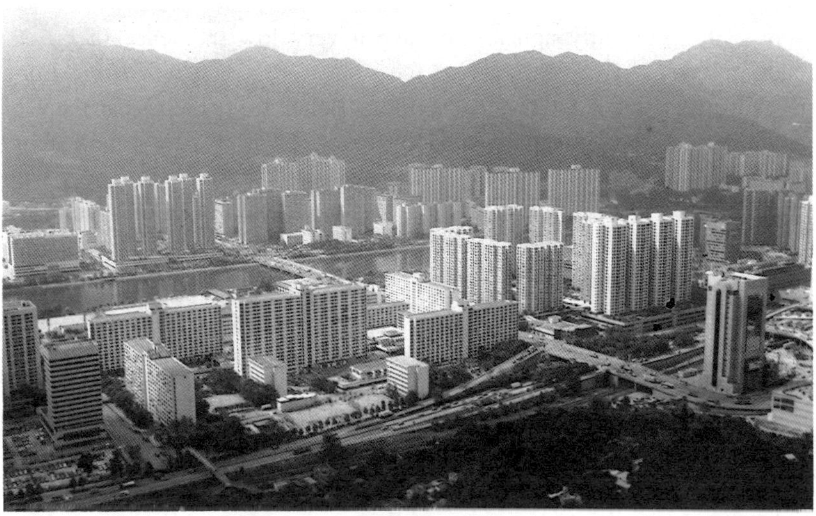

of which seems to be fading away as the pressure on needs to accommodate an increasing population have to be met. Huge new townships are being built on land reclaimed from the sea and previous agricultural areas. Sha Tin, where we are now, is such a township (Figure 1) with a current estimated population of about 600,000. The population of Hong Kong is close to six million of who about 98% are ethnic Chinese. Rapid and extensive improvements over the past couple of decades in housing, medical care, care of the pregnant mother and her baby, overall improved financial well-being, better nutrition and immunization have resulted in infant mortality falling from 61/1,000 in 1966 to 7.5/1,000 in 1987. The pattern of illness in childhood now bears close similarities with those in other developed parts of the world.

Dietary Practices

No territory-wide survey has been carried out to determine the current pattern of food intake during infancy throughout Hong Kong. What is known must be gleaned from various small studies which have been undertaken along with some unwritten opinion.

Breast-feeding

Hong Kong currently appears to have a very low incidence of breast-feeding. Twenty-five years ago in the study *Growing Up in Hong Kong* by Professor Elaine Field and Dr. Flora Baber from the Department of Paediatrics of the University of Hong Kong, 34% of a sample of about 700 babies were being wholly breast-fed for the first 6 months with another 24% partially breast-fed over this time.[1] Recent studies from Sha Tin in the New Territories describe a dramatically changed scene since this time. Wong and his colleagues[2] show that of 256 mothers delivered normally in the Prince of Wales Hospital (102 primiparous, 154 multiparous) serving a relatively low-income group in Sha Tin New Town, only 27%, when interviewed on arrival at the postnatal ward, expressed a wish to breast-feed. What of the outcome in these initially motivated mothers? An answer can be found in another study from Sha Tin from our own department, and one to which I will refer in more detail later, where 174 babies attending a low-cost public housing estate MCH clinic have been followed for their growth and nutrient status. Of 24% breast-feeding at 7 days, only 8, 6 and 2% respectively were still breast-feeding at 2, 4 and 6 months.[3] Figure 2 makes some interesting and self-explanatory comparisons with recent breast-feeding statistics from Australia,[4] United Kingdom,[5] and Guangzhou.[6] My discussions with doctors and nurses working in other areas of the territory point to a similar pattern throughout Hong Kong.

I will not dwell on reasons for such a low local incidence of breast-feeding other than mention that the ready availability of milk formulae, a family income which can now afford breast-milk substitutes, misconceptions held by mothers over the value of breast-feeding, the need and desire to return to work soon after delivery, short maternity leave, lack of privacy, poorly motivated doctors and nurses, and a Hong Kong life-style full of urgency and pressure all contribute in their individual ways. In this regard, Hong Kong seems to resemble other large Asian cities where socio-demographic factors act to favour the bottle in preference to the breast. For example, we have heard already in this workshop from Professor Tan a similar story in Singapore. But perhaps not only in Asia.

Figure 2. Breast-feeding in Sha Tin Compared with Recent Data from Australia,[4] England and Wales[5] and Guangdong Province[6] (South China).

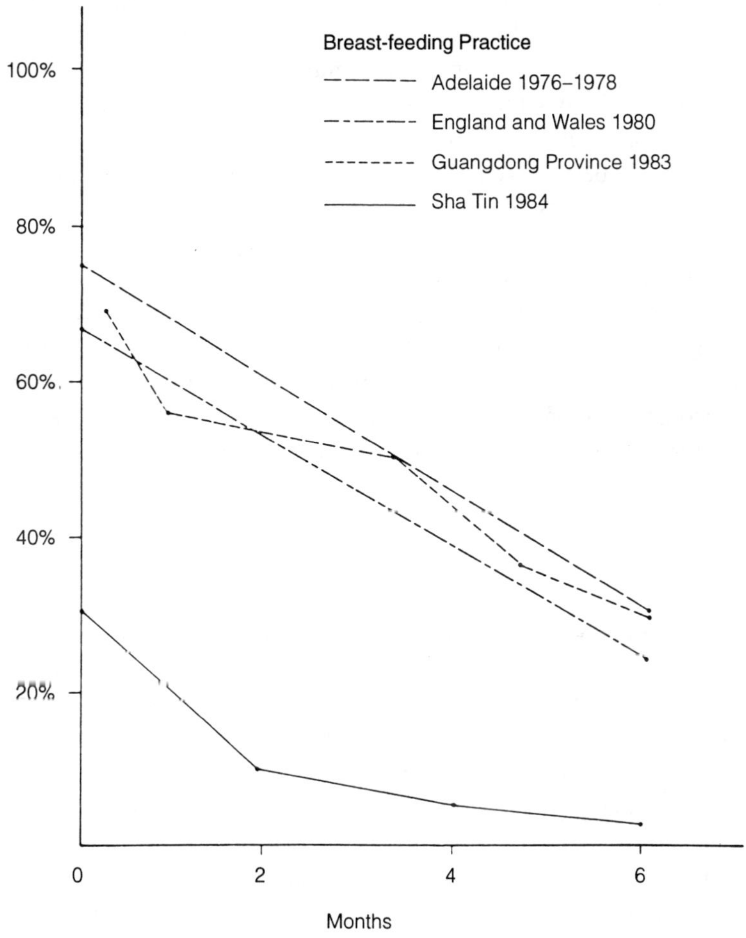

I was interested to read recently of a small nutritional study by Tan and Wheeler in London in 1980[7] where of 20 Chinese babies studied, all but one was bottle-fed. It appears therefore that lifestyle and attitude of Chinese mothers living in comparatively affluent environments are not at the present time conducive to breast-feeding.

Bottle-feeding

What of the milks offered as breast-milk substitutes? In brief, the milks offered are many and varied and reflect Hong Kong's open market policy for the sale of infant formulae.[8] Nearly all comply with international nutritional recommendations.[9] Our own studies in Sha Tin show that at 6 months casein-dominant and whey-dominant formulae were given to 44% and 49% of babies respectively with 3% on soy protein lactose-free formula and 4% on a "follow on" high-protein milk.[8] After 6 months, "follow on" formulae are increasingly being given. What is interesting and important is that our babies from 4 months of age onwards often take less than the recommended volume of milk (Figure 3). This is an important point, especially relevant to those who work in MCH clinics, and it helps to explain many of our mothers' worries that their babies are not fed enough milk. Because weight gain is satisfactory over the first 6 months (see later), we have suggested that manufacturers of various milk formulae should re-examine their recommendations for milk intakes.[3] Without this awareness of a smaller than recommended milk intake in our young infants, attempts will inevitably be made to "force feed," with very undesirable consequences.

Weaning

The introduction of non-milk foods, the beginning of weaning, is between 4–6 months with congee usually the first food.[10,11] Barley and rice water are sometimes used to reconstitute milk powder to help prevent constipation. Iron-fortified cereals are often given initially to begin to accustom babies to the taste and texture of solid foods but rarely are these continued after about 8 months. Meat, fish, fruit, vegetables and eggs will be gradually introduced over the next 6 months or so. The habit of removing meat and fish from the diet (so prevalent in Field and Baber's study),[1] and also described in studies in the early 1980s by Dr. Anita Li and her colleagues in their studies of MCH clinics in Aberdeen and Kwun Tong[10,11] was, in our Sha Tin study, a very unusual practice as also was that reported by Li[10,11] of diluting the milk formula before feeding. The vital message that milk must continue an important food over the weaning period seems now to be heeded with Li describing between 300–500 ml being taken well into the second year.[11] This contrasts with experiences in the 1960s when there was often an abrupt cessation of milk intake once weaning commenced.[1] By

Figure 3. Average Volumes of Full Strength Milk Taken on Day 7 and at 2, 4 and 6 Months[3] by a Sample of Hong Kong Babies.

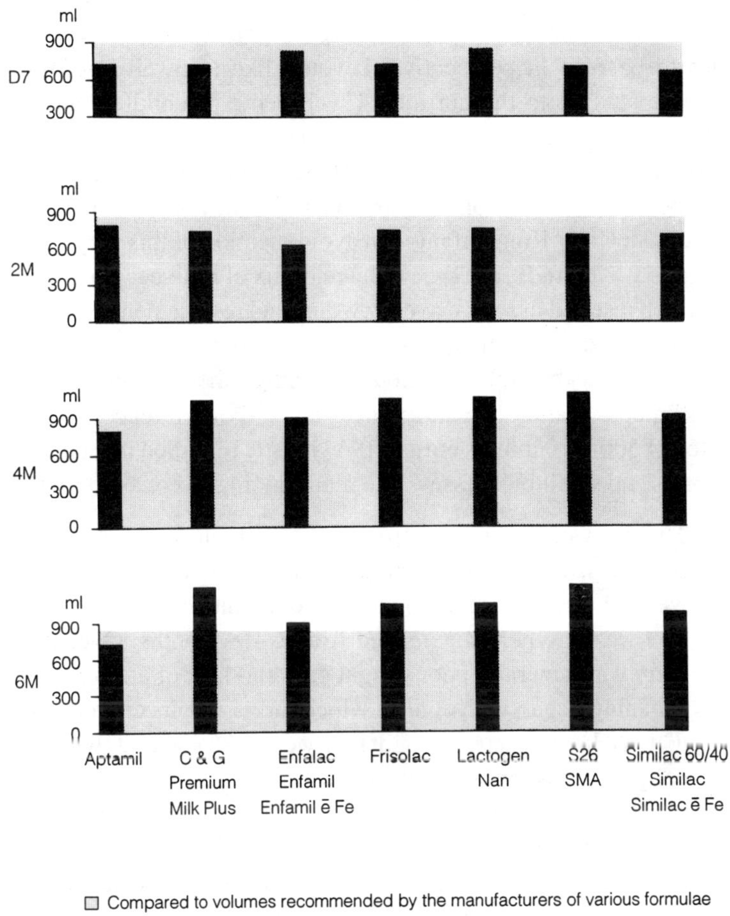

about the age of 24 months, the young child in Hong Kong is now taking "mini" adult diet.

Does the Diet Satisfy Nutritional Requirements?

So much for an overall view of the contemporary pattern of food intake in Hong Kong over the first couple of years of life. I would now like to turn to what is known about the extent to which the young infant diet satisfies optimum nutritional requirements. Because of space, I will limit myself to considerations of iron, calcium, vitamin D, energy and protein intakes.

To set the scene, and to allow the achievements of the last couple of decades to be seen in perspective, I would like to dwell briefly on the prospective study into the nutritional well-being of children, along with their development and rearing practices that was conducted 25 years ago by Professor Elaine Field and Dr. Flora Baber[1] and to which reference has already been made. No commentary on the nutritional adequacy of the current diet in Hong Kong infants can avoid mention of this very important investigation. The study, at a time of huge influx of refugees from mainland China which resulted in severe overcrowding and resettlements estates being rapidly erected to accommodate the increase in population, was promoted by a concern that the children, though looking otherwise in good health, were still much smaller than an English standard of reference. The sample consisted of 500–700 infants born in 1967 mostly to skilled manual workers in factories and small businesses. The main findings were as follows:

1. The pre-weaning period from birth to about 6 months posed few problems, with weight gain adequate and health very good. 50% were wholly or partially breast-fed over this time.
2. The weaning period extended from 6–18 months. Over this time there was generally poor weight gain and lack of arm muscle bulk. Weaning began with congee which largely replaced milk from the diet. A lot of the meat and fish were often withdrawn from the congee, being considered indigestible for small infants. Making matters worse were the many respiratory tract infections suffered and which further reduced food intake and stretched metabolic demands. The picture painted of the weanling was one of lethargy, listlessness and flabby; "a picture of protein calorie malnutrition." But by about 2 years of age immunity had lessened the impact of infection, diet was improved and an "adult diet" was taken.

Strongly worded recommendations emerged out of this study: (1) a more detailed survey of the weaning diet was called for; (2) a greater variety of foods needed to be introduced at a much earlier age soon after weaning had commenced, especially fish, eggs, meat and vegetables; (3) certain foods during illness were not to be withheld; (4) milk should continue to be given throughout the weaning period; (5) environmental improvements to lessen chances of respiratory infections were mandatory. As it will be seen, the improved nutritional state of Hong Kong children has many of its roots in these recommendations.

The next important series of published studies on the state of nutrition during weaning, encouraged by Field and Baber's monograph and an increasing realization throughout the paediatric world of the importance of nutrition for health and well-being in both short and long terms, were undertaken in Aberdeen and Kwun Tong, large townships on Hong Kong Island and the Kowloon Peninsular in the late 1970s and early 1980s by Dr. Anita Li and her colleagues.[10,11] At first sight, however, these studies, of Cantonese babies, were to suggest that surprisingly little had changed since the 1960s.

These cross-sectional studies were of babies brought for routine follow-up visits to the family health clinics for immunization and developmental screening between 7 and 24 months. A total of 180 babies were examined, measured and had their dietary intakes taken on the occasion using 24-hour recall backed up by food checks. Findings in the two studies were very similar and I shall use the second and more comprehensive study from Kwun Tong (9 infants aged between 7–12 months, 47 between 12–18 months and 24 between 18–24 months old) as my reference. Its major conclusions were:

1. 74% of diets had a caloric intake below the 1974 recommended dietary allowance (RDA).[12]
2. 19% had a protein intake less than the RDA.
3. Physical growth suggested undernutrition in 20%.
4. Intakes of iron were unsatisfactory in about 48%; calcium in 54%; vitamin D in 99%; (excluding supplements) vitamin B complexes in about 70% and vitamin C in 67%.

Explanations offered for these nutritional inadequacies centred around the extensive and prolonged use of congee with its low energy content and resulting insufficient intake of milk, which was often offered in dilute form. A reported common practice in 20% of mothers was also the removal of meat and fish particles from congee on account of their apparent indigestibility, thereby losing a valuable source of iron and protein. The authors further inferred that this poor weaning diet was likely to be prevalent throughout Hong Kong.

These studies painted a rather gloomy picture of surprisingly little change since the 1960s. The written media also became a little carried away with the problem with the following headline from one of our main English language newspapers in August 1983 — "HK Babies Go Hungry, Say Studies." The article continued, "about one fifth of Hong Kong babies are severely undernourished in the crucial period between the ages of seven months and two years."[13] That some infants might have been underfed I do not doubt but I wonder, with the benefit of hindsight, if some of the claims were slightly exaggerated, especially when stating that the pattern of nutritional inadequacies were also likely to be prevalent for the whole of Hong Kong. I offer five reasons for my reservations.

1. The RDA for energy is used as a reference from the 1974 recommendations.[12] The recently published 1985 FAO/WHO/UNO recommendations[14] have adjusted these energy allowances, after taking into account studies from England,[15] Sweden[16] and Canada[17] to a 10–15% reduction in energy requirements between 6–12 months. The energy intake reported in Li's study might in this light therefore appear more respectable. At this stage, we would also do well to remind ourselves of the definition of RDA. These are simply mathematically derived levels of specific nutrient intakes that are considered on existing scientific information of the day, to be adequate for practically all populations under consideration. The following statement from the 1985 recommendations is an apt summary of the reasons why the RDA should not be uncritically applied. "A remarkable feature of the reports that emerge is the way in which the emphasis and sometimes the figures change from one meeting to the next.... However the main reason is that at each meeting new areas of ignorance are defined and this stimulates research." Furthermore, the RDA only very occasionally refers to "average" amounts. For energy the RDA is the average of individual requirements, but for other nutrients such as protein, iron, calcium and vitamin D, the RDA is more a safe level of intake — an amount to meet or even exceed the requirements of practically all individuals in a particular group. This safe level is usually obtained by calculating the mean requirement and adding an amount of two standard deviations above this value. Children might therefore have a specific nutrient intake below their RDA yet still have sufficient for their needs.

2. In the dietary calculations, the 50th centile for weight for age was used and not the existing body weight. This already presumes underweight for age and exaggerates any inadequacy in relation to the RDA.
3. A very low oral vitamin D intake is not surprising in subtropical climates and should not conceal the fact that the major potential source of this vitamin is from the action of sunlight, an abundance of which is to be found in Hong Kong, on cholesterol esters in the skin.
4. The babies studies were aged 7–24 months and were considered altogether. This is too wide an age group to allow precise judgements on the adequacy of nutrient intake over such a length of time by nutritional needs, and hence intakes might be expected to vary considerably.
5. Single measurements of weight and height are, I believe, insufficient to make pronouncement that 74% of infants were having an inadequate energy intake for their growth needs.

For these reasons, it is my contention that the general view expressed of the weaning diet was a little too pessimistic. Notwithstanding, these studies served a very important purpose in awakening us to the fact that much had still to be learned about the weaning diet in Hong Kong. As a new arrival to Hong Kong at that time, I was viewing a rather strange paradox: young infants who looked to me to be remarkably healthy yet were being written about as suffering a not inconsiderable degree of occult undernutrition. Through generous support of the Croucher Foundation, we therefore embarked on an investigation to learn more about the nutritional adequacy of both pre-weaning and weaning diets, on this occasion in Sha Tin New Town, a new urban development in the New Territories (Figure 1). A total of 174 babies were recruited at random at an average age of 7 days in a low-cost housing estate MCH clinic in 1984. They have subsequently been seen at 2-monthly intervals for the first year, and 3-monthly thereafter when detailed information on their nutrient intake (collected by 24-hour recall), health and growth have been collected by a research team constituting a dietitian, nurse as well as a paediatrician. This study is beginning to provide some valuable information which improves our understanding of the quantity and quality of nutrient intakes in early childhood and in particular casting some doubts on assumptions of dietary inadequacies. I will briefly summarize some of our findings to date.

Pre-weaning Period: Birth to 6 Months

Energy intake very closely follows the 1985 RDA[14] and other recent reports[15–17] (Table 1). Weight gain closely follows, and sometimes "betters" the NCHS[18] reference standard (Figure 4). Of interest to this meeting are remarkable similarities with weight gain in Dr. Whitehead's Cambridge

Table 1. Mean Daily Energy Intake (kcal/kg) in about 150 Hong Kong Chinese Infants over the First 6 Months Compared with Other Reports.

Age (month)	Present study	Whitehead[15] (1981)	Persson[16] (1984)	Dewey[17] (1983)	FAO/WHO/ UNO[14] (1985)	FAO/WHO[12] (1973)
0.5	121 (7 days)	115	—	113 (1m)	124	120
2	109	102	—	105	114	120
4	88	90	—	93	101	110
6	85	85	87	89	95	110

Figure 4. The Mean Weight Curves of Sha Tin (Hong Kong) Boys and Girls (——) over the First 6 Months Plotted on the NCHS Reference Grid (- - - -).[18]

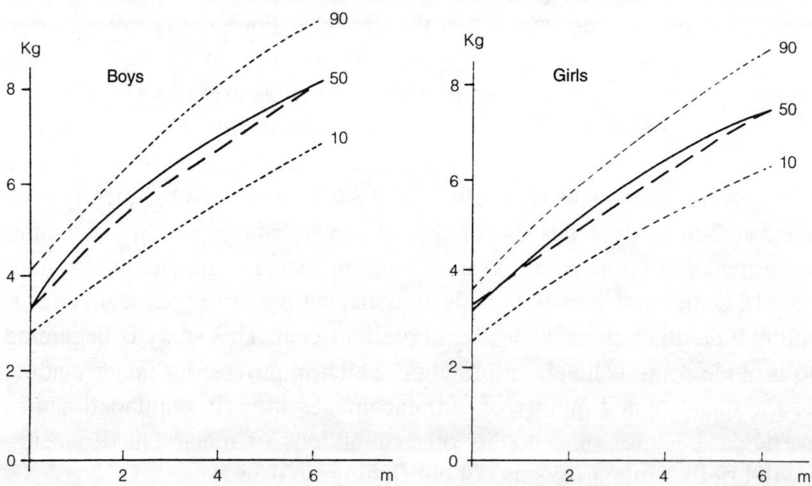

Figure 5. Mean Weights of Sha Tin (Hong Kong) (-●-) and Cambridge (-○-) Boys and Girls from Birth to 6 Months, Expressed as Percentage of the 50th Percentile of the NCHS Reference.[18]

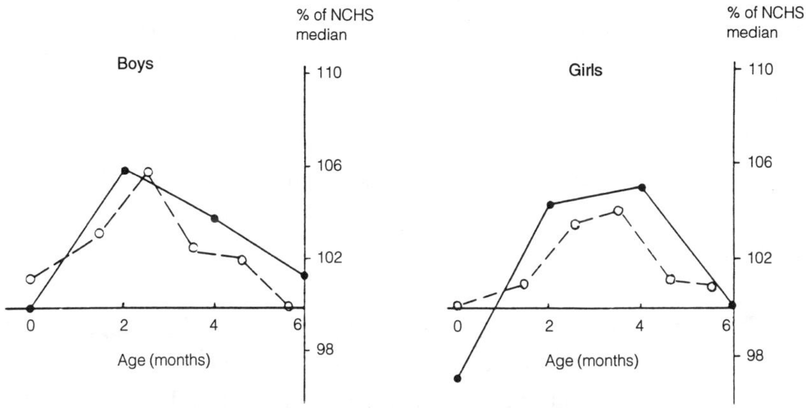

babies most of whom were breast-fed (Figure 5).[19] Thus, even with such low rates of breast-feeding — 24% at birth, 8%, 6% and 3% at 2, 4 and 6 months as previously mentioned — there appear to be no immediate problems for early growth. However, there were 44 episodes of gastroenteritis experienced by these children. Might these have been reduced had more babies been breast-fed?

Weaning Period: 6–24 Months

Iron Status

Iron deficiency is probably the most common single nutrient deficiency worldwide during weaning due to the rapid growth of infants and often inadequate diet at a time when iron stores laid down in prenatal life are progressively consumed.[20] In many poor countries, the reported incidence of iron deficiency over the weaning period is in the order of 40–80%.[21] Even socially advantaged countries have not escaped. In the United Kingdom for example, recent studies have described incidences of between 12% and 45%,[22,23] with children of parents from the Indian subcontinent being especially at risk. Iron deficiency in these young children is mainly dietary, reflecting an inadequate intake during the weaning period through consumption of fresh cow's milk (which can cause occult intestinal blood loss) and weaning foods insufficient in iron.

Table 2 summarizes iron intake (together with ascorbic acid because of its facilitating action on iron absorption) from birth to 18 months in our study in relation to haemoglobin, mean corpuscular volume (MCV) and serum ferritin.[24] Daily iron intake was comfortably within the WHO's RDA of 5–10 mg.[25] Mean haemoglobin was 12.4 g/dl. Eleven infants had a haemoglobin concentration of 11 gm/dl. Of these 7 had β-thalassaemia trait; 2 showed a satisfactory response to iron therapy (2 mg/kg/day); one had an unchanged haemoglobin and one defaulted further follow-up. Mean serum ferritin at 18 months in 128 infants was 155.9 mg/ml. Only one had a concentration < 7 ug/ml.

This very low (2% excluding β-thalassaemia trait) incidence of iron deficiency we attribute to infant feeding practices which provide: (1) an adequate iron intake during the weaning period from milk formula, iron-fortified cereals, meat and fish; and (2) negligible consumption of pasteurized cow's milk with its low iron content and risk of causing occult intestinal blood loss. These findings strongly contrast with those in the Kwun Tong/Aberdeen study[10,11] where about 40% were considered to have insufficient iron intake.

Table 2. Iron Status of about 150 Hong Kong Chinese Infants from 6–18 Months. Mean Values (SD).

Age	Daily intakes		Haemoglobin (gm/dl)	MCV (fl)	Serum ferritin (ng/ml)
	Iron (mg)	Ascorbic acid (mg)			
6m (n=154)	8 (5)	57 (23)	—	—	—
12m (n=155)	9 (3)	61 (27)	—	—	—
18m (n=152)	8 (3)	58 (36)	12.4 (9) (n=123)	77 (7) (n=123)	156 (25) (n=128)
RDA	5–10 mg	20 mg			

Source: Modified from Leung, *et al.*, 1988.[24]

Calcium and Vitamin D

These nutrients I consider as "chemical markers" for the homeostasis of bone mineralization, the nearest we can get to "composition" of skeletal growth. Table 3 shows calcium and vitamin D intakes from milk and other dairy foods at 6, 12, 18 and 24 months in our infants. Other than at 6 months, calcium intakes compare more than favourably with the RDA — which to stress again is a *safe level* of intake. Vitamin D intakes are less than the customary 400 I.U. (10 ug) recommended, but this, it must be remembered, is an empirical estimate based on no very firm scientific data. It must also not be forgotten that a major source of vitamin D is obtained from the action of sunlight on cholesterol precursors in the skin. The RDA makes little or no allowance for this in tropical and subtropical regions. The minimum amount of vitamin D needed to maintain normal mineral homeostasis in the presence of adequate sunlight is not known. However, the FAO/WHO expert group admits that part of all the 400 I.U. might well be supplied through exposure to sunlight.[25] Plasma 25(OH)D3 is a useful marker for the availability to the bones of vitamin D. Figure 6 shows plasma levels in 123 babies at 18 months. In only one was a concentration below 10 ug/ml, the lower limit of the acceptable range.[23]

I conclude from these data that calcium intake over the weaning period is adequate for the needs of the growing skeleton. The normal vitamin D

Table 3. Daily Calcium and Vitamin D Intake in about 150 Hong Kong Chinese Infants between 6–24 Months. Mean Values (SD).

Age	Calcium (mg)	Vitamin D (I.U.)
6m (n=154)	463 (176)	335 (121)
12m (n=155)	598 (283)	261 (107)
18m (n=154)	716 (301)	205 (128)
24m (n=147)	760 (421)	189 (156)
RDA	500 mg	400 I.U.

Source: Unpublished data.

Figure 6. 25 Hydroxycholecalciferol in 123 Hong Kong Chinese Infants Aged 18 Months.

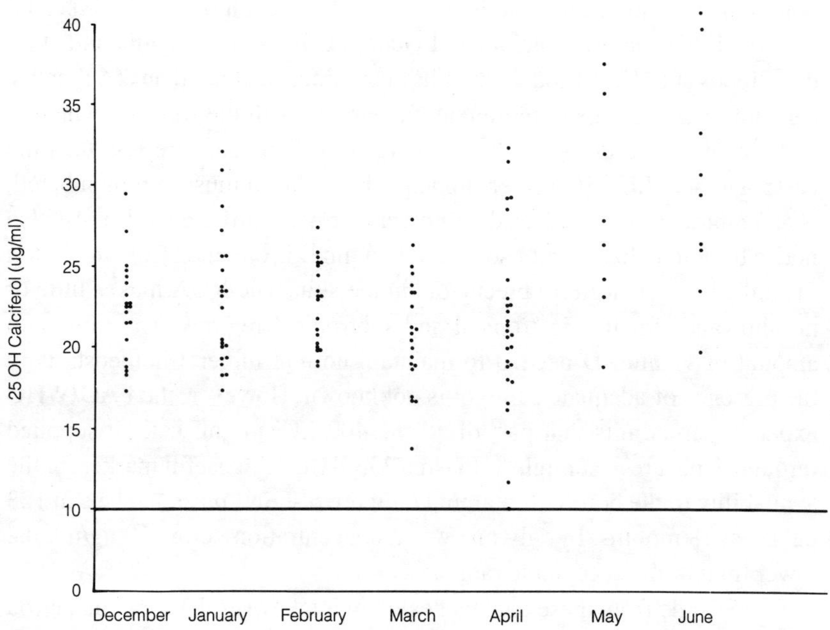

levels in plasma also provide no evidence of any nutritional inadequacy of this vitamin so essential for skeletal growth. This inference receives further support from general paediatric clinical experience in Hong Kong where clinical dietary rickets is now accepted to be exceedingly rare.

Protein/Energy Intake and Physical Growth

The usual clinical marker for adequacy of protein/energy intake is physical growth, hence the reason for considering these three elements together.

Figure 7 shows three examples of mean curves of longitudinal growth of our babies against the NCHS reference curves,[18] the references currently recommended by WHO for international use, in our Sha Tin sample. For weight, length and head circumference the pattern is similar, with deviation away from the reference median between 6 and 12 months. Does this deviation indicate an overall failure of growth and protein/energy insufficiency? I do not believe it does.

Figure 7. Weight in Girls and Head Circumference and Length in Boys. Mean Curves of Sha Tin Babies, about 75 of Each Sex, Compared with the NCHS Reference.[18]

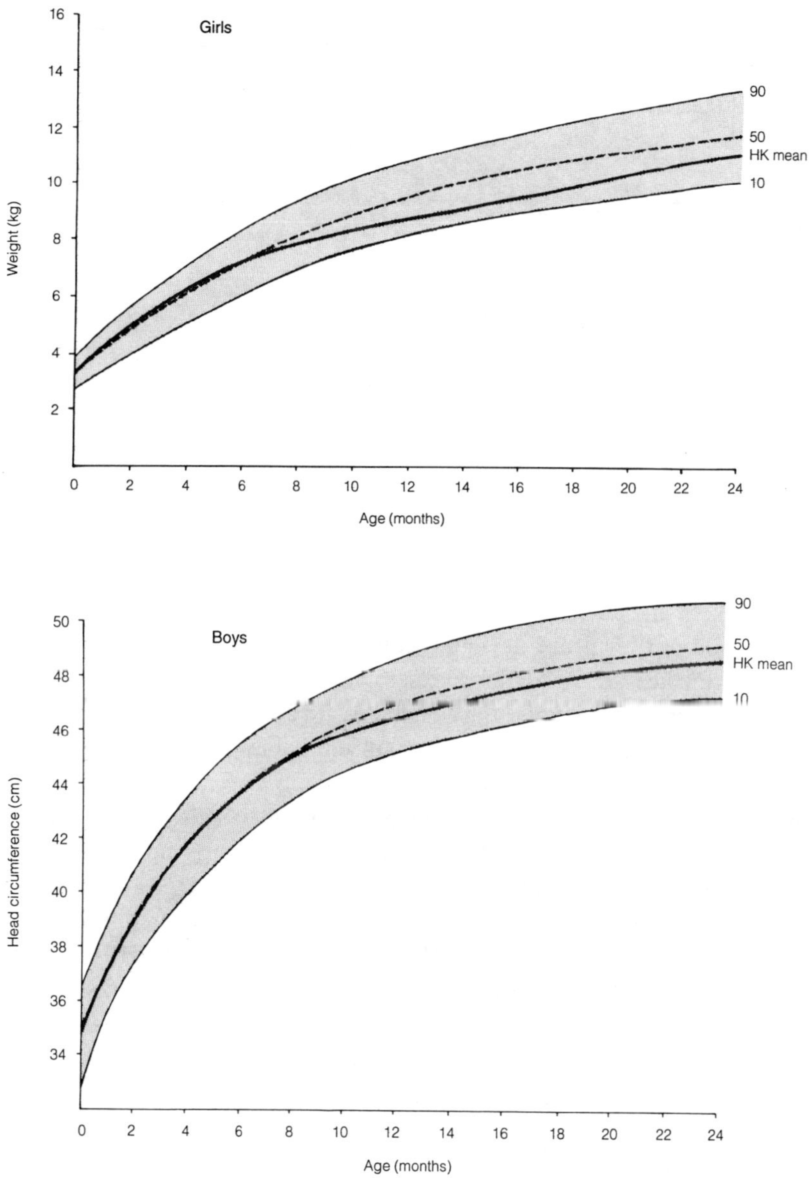

Figure 7. (Cont'd)

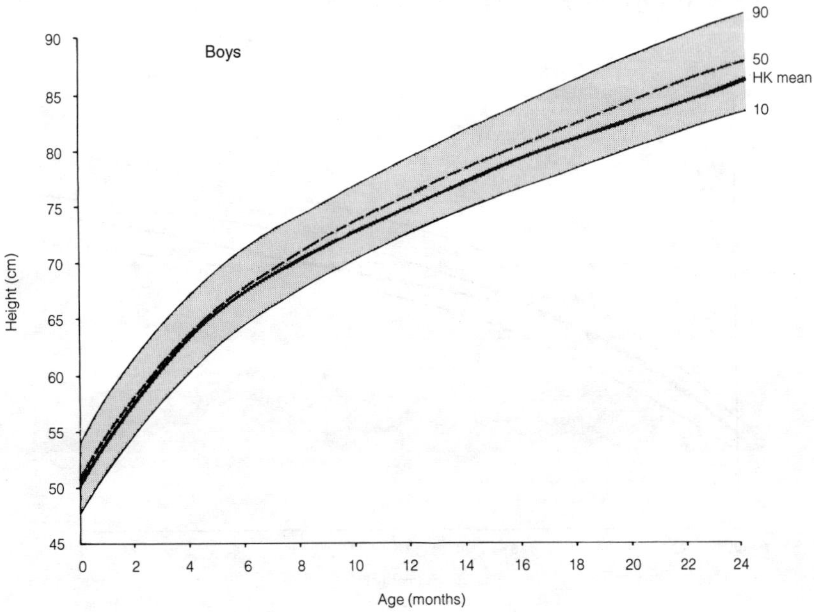

Protein and energy intakes are shown in Table 4. Energy intakes over the period of downward deviation compared favourably with the RDA.[14] Protein intakes are if anything excessive. Thus, because (1) the overall pattern of growth is similar for weight, length and head circumference, i.e. proportionate deviation; (2) as a group the babies enjoyed overall good health; and (3) their iron, calcium and vitamin D status was remarkably good, I do not believe that the growth of our babies is less than adequate. The corollary to this is therefore that protein and energy intakes are satisfactory. I hold the view, already argued,[26] that the "faltering" growth profile represents more a different pattern of growth when compared with that of children of European origin and who largely make up the NCHS reference. The 1985 Joint FAO/WHO/UNO on this aspect states "... that young children of different ethnic groups should be considered as having the same or similar growth potential."[14] I disagree, especially when the growth under question is that of Asiatic children who as a group show definite downward deviation from their NCHS reference mean.[26] This all begs the question of what is satisfactorily growth ... but that surely is another question!

Table 4. Daily Energy and Protein Intakes from 6–24 Months in 150 Hong Kong Chinese Babies. Mean Values (SD).

Age	Energy (kcal/kg)	RDA (average requirement)	Protein (g/kg)	RDA (safe intake)
6m (n=158)	83 (23)	95	2.2 (0.9)	1.7
12m (n=156)	98 (25)		4.7 (1.9)	1.5
18m (n=154)	98 (28)	107	4.8 (1.6)	1.2
24m (n=147)	91 (26)		4.3 (1.4)	

Source: Unpublished data.

Conclusion

This preliminary examination of our data offers encouraging findings that, in our population at least, there is no evidence for clinically important undernutrition. The lessons of the past seem to be heeded. But whether we can extrapolate these findings to the whole of Hong Kong I leave it to you to judge. I will venture that we can, although I do not doubt that as in all big cities, there exist pockets of undernutrition. Firstly, our babies were fed according to guidelines provided and widely implemented in the 47 MCH clinics in the first couple of years. Secondly, in Hong Kong there is a very good attendance at these MCH clinics in the first couple of years. Thirdly, as judged by the type of housing of their parents, the babies are "socially comparable" with Hong Kong as a whole. For those in the audience who doubt these conclusions, I ask one favour. Please investigate and report the nutritional status in your particular group of children!

I will not discuss concerns of overnutrition and obesity. That we see fat babies cannot be doubted but whether too many depends very much on our criteria for obesity. Our study was initially set up to investigate the possibilities of undernutrition. The data will in time be examined to determine whether or not obesity is emerging as a problem.

There is further room for optimism about our infant's food intake. If the weaning diet is analysed for its fat, protein and carbohydrate proportions, we find a major difference with the Western infants' weaning diet having a significantly lower fat content with only 30% of energy intake (unpublished data). If this pattern of nutrient intake continues into adulthood, then this might well reduce one of the risk factors for degenerative vascular disease. This argument of course does not take into account one very important factor, namely the very low incidence of breast-feeding. Professor David Barker in this symposium has already hinted that this might be an important influence in increasing vulnerability in adult years to the premature onset of ischaemic heart disease. Perhaps this should add a damper to our optimism. What it does highlight, however, is the need always to consider in the long term our quest to determine optimum nutrition in infancy and early childhood. It is now insufficient to consider only short-term benefits.

Acknowledgements

I would like to thank my colleagues Dr. S. F. Leung, Mrs. L. Lo and Miss S. Lui, who are conducting the prospective study on Sha Tin babies allowing me a preliminary examination of their findings; Dr. David Leung for helping in the early computerization of the data; The Croucher Foundation for the generous funding of the study; and Miss Juliet Lee for her patience and tolerance in the preparation of this manuscript.

References

1. Field, C. E., and Baber, F. M. *Growing Up in Hong Kong*. Hong Kong: Hong Kong University Press, 1973.
2. Wong, F.W.S., Chow, J.K.K., Loong, E.P.L., *et al.* Attitudes and Knowledge of Mothers Concerning Breast-feeding in a Suburban Population in Hong Kong. *J HK Med Assoc*, 1986; 38:77–87.
3. Leung, S.S.F., Lui, S., Lo, L., *et al.* A Reevalution of Volume of Milk and on Energy Intake of Bottle-fed Babies in the First Six Months. *J HK Med Assoc*, 1988; 38:171–74.
4. Boulton, T.J.C., and Coote, L. M. Nutritional Studies during Early Childhood II. Feeding Practices during Infancy, and Their Relationship to Socio-economic and Cultural Factors. *Aust Paediatr J*, 1979; 15:81–86.
5. *Infant Feeding*, 1980. Office of Population Censuses and Surveys, Social Survey Division, No. 21. London: HMSO, 1982.

6. 楊瑞文、崔燕薇、曾承琬：〈廣東省五市 0-6 月齡嬰兒母乳餵養情況調查〉。發表於一九八五年中華醫學會廣東分會兒科第八屆學術會議。
7. Tan, S. P., and Wheeler, E. F. Food Intakes and Growth of Young Chinese Children in London. *Comm Med*, 1980; 2:20–24.
8. Leung, S.S.F., and Davies, D. P. A Guide through the Jungle of Infant Milk Formulae. *The Hong Kong Practitioner*, 1985; 7(6):1,346–53.
9. Codex Alimentarius Commission. Recommended International Standards for Foods for Infants and Children. Food and Agriculture Organization of the United Nations. *Joint FAO/WHO Food Standards Programme*, 1976; CAC/RS/72/74.
10. Li, A.M.C., Baber, F. M., and Leung, V. S. A Pilot Study on the Weaning Diets of Hong Kong Children. *J HK Med Assoc*, 1982; 34:87–92.
11. Li, A.M.C., Baber, A.F.M., Yu, A.M.C., *et al.* The Weaning Diet of Hong Kong Children. *J HK Med Assoc*, 1985; 37(4):167–75.
12. World Health Organization. Energy and Protein Requirements. Report of a Joint FAO/ WHO *ad hoc* Expert Committee. *WHO Technical Report Series*, No. 522. Geneva: WHO, 1973.
13. *South China Morning Post*, 7 August 1983.
14. World Health Organization. Energy and Protein Requirements. Report of a Joint FAO/WHO/UNO Meeting. *WHO Technical Report Series*, No. 724. Geneva: WHO, 1985.
15. Whitehead, R. G., Paul, A. A., and Cole, T. J. A Critical Analysis of Measured Food Energy Intake during Infancy and Early Childhood in Comparison with Current International Recommendations. *J Hum Nutr*, 1981; 35:339–48.
16. Persson, L. A., Johansson, E., and Samuelson, G. Dietary Intake of Weaned Infants in Swedish Community. *Hum Nutr: App Nutr*, 1984; 38A:247–54.
17. Dewey, K. G., and Lonnerdal, B. Milk and Nutrient Intake of Breast-fed Infants from 1 to 6 Months: Relation to Growth and Fatness. *J Pediatr Gastroenterol Nutr*, 1983; 3:497.
18. United States, Public Health Service, Health Resources Administration. NCHS Growth Charts. *Rockville, M.D.*, 1976; HRA 76 1120,23,3.
19. Whitehead, R. G., and Paul, A. A. Growth Charts and the Assessment of Infant Feeding Practices in the Western World and in Developing Countries. *Early Hum Dev*, 1984; 9:187–207.
20. Vyas, D., and Chandra, R. K. Functional Implications of Iron Deficiency. In Steckel, A., ed., *Iron Nutrition in Infancy and Childhood.* New York: Nestle, Vevey/Raven Press, 1984; 45–59.
21. Florentino, R. F., and Guirriec, R. M. Prevalence of Nutritional Anaemia in Infancy and Childhood with Emphasis on Developing Countries. Ibid., 61–72.
22. Ehrhardt, P. Iron Deficiency in Young Bradford Children from Different Ethnic Groups. *BMJ*, 1986; 292:90–93.

23. Grindulis, H., Scott, P. H., Belton, N. R., *et al.* Combined Deficiency of Iron and Vitamin D in Asian Toddlers. *Arch Dis Child*, 1986; 61:843–48.
24. Leung, S.S.F., Davies, D. P., Lui, S., *et al.* Iron Deficiency Is Uncommon in Healthy Hong Kong Infants at 18 Months. *J Trop Paed*, 1988; 34:100–3.
25. World Health Organization. Requirements of Ascorbic Acid, Vitamin D, Vitamin B_{12}, Folate and Iron. Report of a Joint FAO/WHO Expert Group. *WHO Technical Report Series*, No. 452. Geneva: WHO, 1970.
26. Davies, D. P. The Importance of Genetic Influences on Growth in Early Childhood with Particular Reference to Children of Asiatic Origin. In Waterlow, ed., *Linear Growth Retardation in Third World Countries*. Nestle Nutrition Workshop No. 14. New York: Raven Press, Medical and Scientific Publishers, 1988.

4

Early Childhood Nutritional Problems in the Far East: A Commentary

The Hong Kong Journal of Paediatrics, 1988; 5:1–6

The nutrition of infants and young children continues to attract a wide array of professional interest the world over. Yet many problems remain and in these, countries in the Far East are no exception. To name but a few, concern to varying degrees is regularly expressed over a falling overall incidence of breast-feeding; availability of suitable breast-milk substitutes; nutritional inadequacies during weaning and the contribution these elements make to protein/energy malnutrition, vitamin and iron deficiencies; growth failure, diarrhoea and acute respiratory infections, the major contributors to death and serious morbidity of childhood. In more developed areas, complacency is not being allowed to be developed as the low incidence of breast-feeding and increasing adoption of Western-type weaning diets are being paralleled by newly emerging problems of obesity and allergic diseases.

The peoples of the Far East share many a common heritage, lifestyle and ethnic origin. In such a distinct ecology, it seemed worthwhile for those with responsibilities for the well-being of young children to meet and exchange ideas on early childhood nutritional problems in their communities. It was with this idea in mind that an international workshop on "Early Childhood Problems in the Far East," jointly hosted by the Department of Paediatrics, The Chinese University of Hong Kong and the Hong Kong Paediatric Society, recently took place at the Prince of Wales Hospital and the Hotel Riverside Plaza, Sha Tin on Saturday and Sunday, 28 to 29 November 1987.

The workshop, which was officially opened by Mrs. Elizabeth Wong, JP, Director of Social Welfare, was generously sponsored by Wyeth International and Wyeth (Hong Kong) Ltd. and its proceedings are published in a supplement to the 1988 edition (Volume 5) of *The Hong Kong Journal of Paediatrics*.[1] The two-day workshop featured initially on the Saturday afternoon four keynote lectures by renowned international specialists to provide an update of current nutritional concepts: Dr. R. G. Whitehead (Director, MRC Dunn Nutrition Unit, Cambridge University, U.K.); Dr. M. Gracey (Director, Princess Margaret Children's Medical Research Foundation, Perth, Australia); Dr. B. A. Wharton (Consultant Paediatrician, Sorrento Maternity Hospital, Birmingham, U.K.); and Professor D.J.P. Barker (Director, MRC Environmental Epidemiology Unit, University of Southampton, U.K.). The Sunday included 30-minute papers describing current nutritional problems in ten countries/regions in the Far East from invited speakers, all with a special interest in infant nutrition: Dr. S. T. Chen (Malaysia), Professor C. L. Chen (Taiwan), Dr. T. Li (China), Professor S. Ocampo (the Philippines), Professor D. P. Davies (Hong Kong), Dr. Soetjiningsih (Indonesia) and Professor K. S. Chung (Korea). The workshop concluded with a very interesting and often provocative discussion on issues raised during the meeting between the audience and invited speakers.

With such a huge geographical area represented in the workshop, and without participation of some of the poorer countries (Burma, Vietnam, Kampuchea and Laos), it would be naive to even suggest that coverage of the state of childhood nutrition in the region could offer anything other than a very superficial glimpse into the true realities. Notwithstanding, the participants must be thanked for having so painstakingly researched their own problems so that all in the audience could not have failed to leave the workshop without their eyes having been opened and horizons widened to new knowledge.

The importance of adequate maternal nutrition during gestation to allow a well-nourished baby to emerge into the extra-uterine environment, well-equipped to feed from the breast or bottle and able to cope with potential infective environmental insults, was emphasized by Professor K. L. Tan (Singapore). The higher low birth-weight rates in Indonesia, the Philippines, Malaysia and Thailand, with their associated increases in infant mortality and morbidity provide a timely reminder of this important principle. But attention to the mother's diet should not stop at birth. Successful lactation, and on which survival of so many babies in poorer countries demands, also demands adequate nutrition of the mother throughout the extero-gestate fetal stage of development.

The pre-weaning period is characterized by very variable rates of breast-feeding in the region. Especially in Japan and newly industrialized Taiwan, Singapore, Hong Kong and Korea, lifestyle and opportunities provided for working mothers to be economically productive "instead of being merely involved in reproduction" (Tan), and increased prosperity from industrial development which allows purchase of nutritionally adequate approved milk formulae has led to breast-feeding being now much less popular.

In Hong Kong, for example, a recent study gave a 24% incidence at birth falling to 2% at 6 months. There was also consensus that, at least in the near term, much change is unlikely in spite of educational campaigns in these countries to promote breast-feeding. This, as Dr. Gracey commented, contrasts with the current situation in many Western industrialized countries which in recent years have "rediscovered breast-feeding." In his Perth study for example, 25% were still breast-feeding at 12 months. The argument for "emotional nutrition," breast-feeding being used to improve the psychological bonding between mother and baby, a point raised by Dr. Victor Ho (Hong Kong) in the discussion, appears at present to be falling on infertile soil. Whether, as Professor S. Ocampo (the Philippines) prompted, the increasing concern about child abuse and the "new morbidity" of paediatric behavioural disturbances in the more developed parts of the region where family ties, traditionally so strong, have prevented this problem in the past but now showing increasing signs of weakening, will enhance awareness of the importance of breast-feeding remains to be seen. Current realities are that for as long as very low infant mortality rates (among the lowest in the world) parallel falling breast-feeding rates in these newly industrialized countries, little change can be expected.

However, as Dr. Chen (Malaysia) so rightly pointed out, even in industrialized countries, morbidity from gastrointestinal and respiratory disease is still significantly higher in bottle-fed babies. We should therefore not become too complacent. We should also heed the challenging thesis put forward by Professor Barker (Southampton) of possible associations between the premature onset of middle-age degenerative disease (ischaemic heart disease, stroke, respiratory disorders) and the mode of early feeding. A particularly interesting slant to the breast-feeding debate was put by Dr. Yamashiro (Japan) who drew attention on this occasion to unacceptable *complications* of breast-feeding: vitamin K deficiency haemorrhagic disease (where at least 400 new cases a year diagnosed in

Japan), pollution of human milk with Polychlorinated Bi-phenyl from factory waste, organochlorine pesticides and insecticides, and even vertical transmission of HTLV-1 virus from carrier mother's milk. These are problems which require further definition and resolution. (I have to confess being somewhat surprised to discover that vitamin K prophylaxis is not being widely practised in Japan.)

Nevertheless, put alongside the unacceptable consequences of *not* breast-feeding in other countries in the region, notably Indonesia, the Philippines, Malaysia, Thailand and China (and in these countries especially among the rural poor) where gastroenteritis, respiratory infections and seeds of protein/energy malnutrition are very real problems caused by poor environmental sanitation, and limited economic resources that cannot allow safe and adequate formula feeding, these complications have much less immediate impact. In countries where breast-feeding is essential to provide the best possible chances for survival, it was therefore a matter of concern to discover that customs and traditions will often lead to solid foods (rice gruels, mashed banana, etc.) being given very early on, even in the first few weeks after birth. By weakening the suckling urge, lactation will suffer and at the same time bacterial food contamination is introduced commencing the malnutrition — gastroenteritis vicious cycle. In the same vein, an extremely worrying trend in these countries is, through insidious urbanization, commercial pressures and erosion of traditional values, a decline in breast-feeding with deplorable consequences.

From about 6 months onwards for the next 18 months or so, the milk diet, whether breast or approved formula, becomes increasingly insufficient for growth and maintenance needs. This transition period, when (ideally) increased varieties of solid foods should be introduced until an adult-type diet is achieved, constitutes the weaning period where many nutritional disorders begin to rear their ugly heads — especially protein/energy malnutrition leading to growth failure, and iron and vitamin deficiencies. These are Dr. Wharton's (Birmingham) "ugly sisters" of the Cinderella of weaning. According to Dr. Whitehead (Cambridge), it is to this weaning period that much of future paediatric nutrition research should be directed. These weaning problems were explicitly described in Thailand, Indonesia, China, Malaysia and the Philippines.

In spite of this, several speakers made the important point that when undernutrition occurs, it is not always solely due to primary lack of nutritious foods in the home. Poor-quality protein and low fat and carbohydrate-density foods from traditional gruels of millet, rice, maize etc. provide all too often a nutritionally inadequate monotony that sets the scene for Cinderella's ugly sisters. The problems are further made worse by an inefficient utilization of nutrients resulting from food contamination, infectious diseases (particularly measles), and poor birth spacing which increases maternal demands and cuts short breast-feeding. Concerning the latter, it is now beyond dispute that morbidity in early childhood contributes a vital role to controlling population growth, a problem which in some of the less fortunate parts of our region threatens to worsen already existing socio-economic instability. Even medical instruction is also not without blame. In parts of China for example, as we heard from Dr. Li Tong (Beijing), a zeal to overcome deficiencies of iron as well as vitamins A and D is causing toxic side effects in worrying proportions.

No better example of these complex medical-economic interactions operating during weaning, and which so often have their roots in poverty and its many associations, can be seen than in the newly industrialized regions of the Far East where in one generation, the disorders of weaning have largely disappeared, paralleling rapid socio-economic progress in these countries. But even here the pendulum will not be still! New problems seem now to be emerging — overnutrition, allergies, obesity and their attendant ills and which have their origins in the rich diversity of weaning foods made available through relative affluence.

A marker of this over-abundance is a 2 to 3-fold increase in protein intake which is common in these countries: they would be well advised not to so radically dcpart from traditional weaning diets where, providing milk continues as an important nutrition source throughout weaning, the rice-based diet with appropriate amounts of added meat, fish, vegetables and fruit provide a good balanced intake. There is no reason, however strong commercial pressures might be, to go "overboard" and adopt Western practices of energy-dense feeding which at the same time also increases considerably the fat content of the diet and sow the seeds for later obesity and even perhaps problems of later life. However, we must still see these worries in perspective. It is sad irony that other countries in the region where undernutrition is so common (for example in the Philippines in 1986 where about 20% of the pre-school population are moderately or severely underweight and in the disadvantaged of Malaysia where the prevalence of moderate forms of protein/energy malnutrition ranges from 7–36%) would be envious of some of these dietary excesses. For these countries, it must seem a luxury to be concerned with childhood obesity, allergies and premature onset of middle-age disease when so many of their children fail to live beyond early childhood.

The solution to the many weaning dilemmas in economically less fortunate countries does not alone rest with making available proprietary, and often expensive, weaning foods. An attitude of self-reliance has to be fostered to encourage locally available foods to be made into a palatable and nutritious weaning diet which with milk as a continuing food, breast or formula, will provide a safe and balanced nutrient intake. An example of what can be achieved through these measures was especially well illustrated by Professor Valysasevi (Thailand) who described the development and use of a rice-based weaning food mixed with soya bean, mung bean, ground nuts and sesame seeds. Within 18 months, the percentage of malnourished pre-school children in two villages in Northeast Thailand fell from 55% to 21% after being given such a weaning diet. Areas of the Philippines also recorded a similar experience. One point however must be made clear. The success of these ventures into self-sufficiency cannot rely solely on local initiative and good will. Support by government ministeries (Health, Education, Community Development, etc.) and university institutions is vital for their success. This in turn can be forthcoming only if health of young infants is considered an essential priority in national health programmes. The recent UNICEF annual report[2] gives greater reason for optimism that the health and well-being of young children is now considered a top priority in most countries.

An important recurring theme throughout the workshop was the "quality control" of the weaning diet through regular growth monitoring. A lively debate led to a consensus that the North American-derived NCHS reference growth charts, though widely used and recommended by WHO as an international standard, are probably not a suitable reference standard for Asiatic children who, between about 6 to 18 months, show consistently a deviation of weight, length and head circumferences away from the expected mean curve. That this profile (which is exaggerated in poor countries during weaning) is probably physiological can be deduced by its clear documentation in children from the more affluent regions such as Japan, Hong Kong, Korea, Singapore, Taiwan and in the socially fortunate of Malaysia, China, Indonesia and Thailand. Failure to recognize and appreciate the significance of biological ethnic differences which lead to slightly smaller physical size compared with Caucasians will encourage adoption of unsuitable weaning practices and invite the emergence of obesity.

The revealing diversity of problems of nutritional origin in our large region exposes yet again the huge gap that continues to exist between the children of wealthy and poor nations and between the socially privileged and underprivileged within nations. The resulting toll on human life and suffering is indecent, unnecessary and unacceptable in an age of remarkable technological achievement. In Hong Kong, along with other newly industrialized nations, the financial boom has allowed improved environmental health and the affordability of nutritious foods. In these countries, there are now, realistically, few serious problems in the short term, although the warning from Professor Barker that influences operating in fetal life and early childhood, through possible programming of metabolic processes, might have an important role in determining later disease need to be heeded and further investigated.

For our less fortunate neighbours, much can be done in the anticipation of improvements in socio-economic conditions. Harmful traditions which render successful breast-feeding difficult should be discouraged; breast-feeding must continue to cover the weaning period; nutritious weaning foods wherever possible using natural local resources must be developed and made readily available; levels of education must be raised; improvements in environmental hygiene need to continue to be emphasized; control of infections through immunization, particularly against measles, must continue its already encouraging upward trend to prevent the vicious malnutrition-infection cycle; growth monitoring must be enforced as a measure to detect early on beginnings of growth failure. These are only some examples especially emphasized by the visiting speakers. To help achieve these objectives, there is need for the science and application of nutrition to feature more in undergraduate and postgraduate curricula. We must strive to intensify awareness that good early nutrition is as important a primary preventive measure for illness as is immunization against infectious diseases.

It is to be hoped that the sharing and exchange of so much knowledge in our workshop, along with ideas that will undoubtedly have been generated, will help create greater understanding, empathy and tolerance between countries in the region leading ultimately towards improved health of our children.

References

1. Early Childhood Nutritional Problems in the Far East. *HK J Paediatr*, 1988; 5 (Supplement).
2. Grant, J. P. *The State of the World's Children*. United Nations Children's Fund (UNICEF). Oxford: Oxford University Press, 1988.

5

How Adequate Is Human Milk for Prematurely Born Babies? Diminishing Confidence in a "Sacred Cow"

The Hong Kong Journal of Paediatrics, 1989; 6:140–60

Summary

Optimum nutrition for preterm babies is that which permits satisfactory growth and health in the short term, free from metabolic problems and infection, and in the long term fulfilment of growth and neuro-developmental potential and physical well-being. Until comparatively recently, the long-held assumption was that human milk best provided these requirements. However, studies showing slower growth rates in preterm infants who were fed human milk have provoked a rethink into its nutritional adequacy. This chapter examines the issue.

The composition of the various types of human milk available to the preterm baby is described along with their short-term influences on early growth, body composition, infection, necrotizing enterocolitis and protein allergy as well as long-term effects on physical size and neuro-psychological function. While admitting that human milk will often fail to meet some of the special nutritional needs of small preterm babies, the argument is put forward that as yet insufficient evidence exists to totally discourage its feeding to these babies if it is available. Its antimicrobial properties, potential immunological benefits and possible advantages to body (and brain) composition justify its continued use. Nowhere is this more important than in those parts of the resource-poor world where risks of neonatal infection are extremely high.

In developed regions of the world where the overall incidence of breast-feeding is very low (as in Hong Kong), and where milk formulae appear to satisfy the requirements of preterm babies perfectly well, a dilemma exists. The development of systems to provide human milk for preterm babies in these areas would best await findings of current research which is being conducted in various parts of the world to determine the true value of human milk for these babies.

The Quest for Optimum Nutrition for Preterm Babies

The survival of prematurely born babies has improved dramatically in recent years due to the many advances which have taken place in perinatal care over this period. However, successful management of early cardio-respiratory hazards, the major contributor to early death, often brings with it one very real problem which has its origins in the physiologically un-prepared state of the gastrointestinal tract of these small babies to digest, absorb and assimilate nutrients: how are they to be optimally nourished when, without premature birth, they would have been otherwise fed across the placenta with a physiological blend of nutrients prepared by the mother? Many of these small babies will be sick or extremely immature and need an initial period of parenteral feeding. But in time enteral nutrition has to be established in all who survive. What is this best possible nutrition?

Optimum nutrition for preterm babies may be considered that which permits satisfactory growth and health in the short term (without overtaxing metabolic and excretory capabilities), free from metabolic problems and infection, and in the long term, fulfilment of genetically endowed growth and psychomotor potential and physical well-being. For babies born at term, there can be no doubt about the superiority of human milk to provide these needs on account, above all else, of the high digestibility of its fat, readily utilizable nitrogen and appropriate balance of minerals and electrolytes (all of whose bioavailability are maximized by recently discovered growth modulators in milk) and the presence of an antimicrobial umbrella of immune substances which offer protection against infections, especially of the gastrointestinal tract. For a long time this assumption of the biological superiority of human milk was also held for preterm babies and it was this that motivated, in the early part of this century, the setting up, in maternity hospitals of economically developed countries, of human milk banks with responsibilities to collect, process and administer human milk to babies whose mothers were unable to sustain adequate lactation: human milk for these babies had to be provided by other breast-feeding mothers. Milk banks have since become an integral part of paediatric care in many parts of the world.

Emerging Doubts over the Adequacy of Human Milk

All seemed well until the 1970s when doubts began to emerge over the desirability of donor milk for preterm babies. Studies were revealing slower growth rates in babies who were fed human milk[1,2] and even its anti-microbial benefits were being questioned as the heat applied to donor milk to free it of microbial contamination was found to destroy many of the physiological functions of its specific antimicrobial substances.[3] But these anxieties, it transpired, were not new. Confidence in human milk as the ideal food for preterm babies had been challenged as early as 1919 when, in Germany, Finkelstein questioned the nutritional adequacy of human milk to provide normal growth.[4] Thereafter doubts had intermittently been expressed that human milk might not offer the best nutrition for babies born very early in the third trimester with their unique nutrition and growth requirements.[5,6]

It is, therefore, timely now to pause and re-examine the adequacy of human milk, with its apparent imperfections, for preterm babies. Although currently a matter of little concern in Hong Kong because of such a low incidence of breast-feeding even among normal term babies, it is nonetheless an important biological issue that should be of interest to all who care for new-born babies if for no other reason than that they need to be prepared to respond to questions put to them should the matter ever be raised.

Macro-nutrient Composition of Donor Breast Milk

This re-evaluation of the nutritional adequacy of human milk has to begin with the appreciation that when it is made available, donor human milk for preterm babies will usually be a "mixture" of various types of milk depending upon how it is collected, processed and administered. Unlike formula feeds, its composition is therefore extremely variable.

Types of Milk

Mature Expressed Milk

This is the milk expressed (by hand expression or electric breast pump suction) from the breast after a feed by a mother who is well established in breast-feeding her own normal baby. It is probably the method of collection most widely used in traditional human milk banks. The average composition of this expressed milk, which usually provides reference standard for the composition of approved milk formulae, is given in Table 1.

Table 1. Average Composition of Human Pooled Expressed Milk.[7]

Energy (Kcal/L)	700
(MJ/L)	2.9
Protein (g/L)	10.7
Lactose (g/L)	74
Fat (g/L)	42
Sodium (mmol/L)	6.4
Potassium (mmol/L)	15
Calcium (mmol/L)	8.7
Magnesium (mmol/L)	1.2

Drip Milk

Especially in the United Kingdom, milk banks continue to obtain milk that has "dripped" passively from the non-feeding breast during a feed. This method, however, seems now to have become increasingly less popular with the demonstration over the past ten years or so that drip milk contains only about one half the amount of fat of expressed milk (Table 2).[8–10] Its composition does not otherwise depart much from expressed milk in its other major nutrients and immune substances.[10] With triglyceride as the chief energy source of milk, babies given drip milk will have a much lower energy intake than those fed expressed milk, an effect accentuated even more by the natural fall in fat content that takes place with time post-partum.[10]

Table 2. Average Composition of Pooled Human Drip Milk.[10]

Energy (Kcal/L)	480
(MJ/L)	2.0
Protein (g/L)	10
Lactose (g/L)	65
Fat (g/L)	22
Sodium (mmol/L)	5.5
Potassium (mmol/L)	16.1
Calcium (mmol/L)	6.9
Magnesium (mmol/L)	1.2

Combined Drip and Expressed Milk

Mothers who combine collection of both drip and expressed milk can provide a food which has advantages over drip and expressed milk alone. A greater volume is obtained than if expressed milk solely is collected and the energy content is only very slightly less than that of expressed milk.[11]

The fat content of donor milk has therefore emerged as the most important nutrient determining the adequacy of human milk for preterm babies. However, at this stage it is also important to draw attention to the fact that not only does the quantity of fat depend on the method of collection. Fatty acid composition also shows considerable variation with the fat content of the maternal diet. As more fats from vegetable sources are included in diets, more long-chain polyunsaturated fatty acids (particularly linoleic and linolenic) are found in donor milk.[12] This holds consequences for digestion and utilization of fat as well as on the composition of both storage and structural lipid.

Preterm Milk

This is the term given to milk which mothers who give birth prematurely are able to express themselves. Somewhat surprisingly its composition has only captured the interest of scientists and clinicians in the past couples of decades, paralleling the general rewakening of interest in breast-feeding: before this time little attempt was made to encourage mothers giving birth prematurely to breast-feed, so its composition was not seen to deserve detailed analysis. But since Atkinson and her colleagues[13] in Toronto first described a higher protein content of preterm milk in 1978, many workers have now investigated the nutrient composition of this milk.[14–20] Its overall composition does appear to differ from term milk but there is no general agreement on the extent of these differences, perhaps not surprising with different methods of collection and stages of gestation combining to give a very heterogeneous mixture of human milk preparations for study.

1. **Nitrogen** — Total nitrogen is about 20% higher than in term milk but the amino acid profile is much the same. Its major contributor is protein, although how this is distributed between nutrient and immunological protein classes remains to be better defined. Preterm milk collected in the first five days has been shown to contain much more secretory IgA (SIgA) than term milk.[21,22] The amount of non-protein nitrogen — creatinine, urea, nucleotides, free amino acids, peptides, uric acid, etc. which account for 25% of human milk nitrogen compared with only 5% in cow's milk — is also a matter for debate. Atkinson and colleagues[14] found a larger amount in preterm milk but others have been unable to confirm these findings.[18]
2. **Fat, lactose and energy** — If methods of collection and analysis are uniform, there would appear to be no consistent differences in the fat and lactose content (and therefore the energy value) of preterm and term milk. Preterm milk has however been shown to be richer in cholesterol, phospholipid and long-chain polyunsaturated fatty acids, the biomembrane substrates of milk.[23]
3. **Mineral and electrolytes** — Sodium and chloride concentrations are higher in the early weeks than in mature milk; calcium and phosphate however have only about 75% the concentration.[17,19] Since preterm babies need large amounts of calcium and phosphate to prevent osteopenia in their rapidly growing skeleton, the potential disadvantage to skeletal development of any human milk feeding is evident.
4. **Antimicrobial properties** — Little is known about the antimicrobial properties of preterm milk. Mention has already been made of greater amounts of SIgA.[21,22] Murphy found cells of similar number and ability to kill staphylococci as in term milk.

Interferon production to endotoxin challenge was also greater.[24] In one study, the concentrations of lactoferrin and lysozyme have been shown to be greater in milk of women delivering prematurely.[25]

The physiology of these compositional variations in preterm milk is not understood, but they are likely to relate to the different endocrine milieu of the mother delivering prematurely. Its overall composition is more typical of a prolonged colostral phase and, more by chance than by design, appears better suited to the nutritional needs of the prematurely born baby. Indeed, what is so remarkable is that in spite of being deprived of a sizeable part of the gestational period, and with its preparation for term childbirth, so many mothers giving birth prematurely are still able to produce milk highly nutritious in quality, although of limited volume.

Effects of Processing and Administration on Nutrient Content

Discussion of the nutrient composition of human milk made available to preterm babies cannot be left without mentioning other influences on composition *after* it has been collected by the mother. There is often an assumption that the composition of milk which enters the baby's gastro-intestinal tract is the same as that which is collected from the mother by whatever method. This is far from being the case.

During Pasteurization

Williamson and his colleagues found that fat from boiled and pasteurized milk averaged 62% and 73% respectively that of unheated milk.[26] They speculated this to be due most likely to the destruction of breast-milk bile salt-stimulated lipase (an enzyme extremely heat-sensitive and secreted in high amounts throughout lactation in both preterm and mature milk and considered to play an important role in fat digestion), thereby limiting fat absorption. Protein utilization and lipolysis of milk triglycerides have also been shown to be adversely affected by heat.[27]

During Storage

Low temperature storage prior to administration affects the pattern of free fatty acids with a tendency to convert to less well-absorbed longer-chain polyenoic acids.[27] Storage also affects the cell content since milk cells adhere to the inside of a container, and in this respect glass is worse than plastic.[28]

During Administration

Another adverse influence is the means by which milk is given to the baby. Human milk fat is often left sticking to the walls of delivery tubes, syringe pumps and burettes used in administering milk: up to 35% of the milk energy content can be lost in this way.[29,30] Continuous feeding causes greater loss than bolus feeding and, perhaps not surprisingly, the slower the rate (needed usually for the smallest of babies) the greater the fat loss.[30] Equally disturbing is that nutritional protein and immunoglobulins are also lost in the process of continuous feeding.[30]

It is therefore clearly wasted effort to spend valuable time (and money) in collecting milk of the best possible nutrient and immune content unless similar care is given to minimize loss of essential nutrients during the processing, storage and administration of milk.

Outcome of Feeding Human Milk to Preterm Babies

This brief review of the composition of human milk that might be fed to preterm babies, along with other influences on its nutrient content highlights the great variations in nutrient intake that can occur. To some clinicians, these variations are unacceptable and substantially weaken the argument for feeding any human milk to infants made especially vulnerable through their immature state. Assuming an average dietary calorie requirement for preterm babies of about 120 Kcal/kg/day, a daily volume of about 250 ml/kg of "average" donor human milk would be given to small babies, thus exposing them to considerable iatrogenic risk. Furthermore, the wide compositional variations render very difficult the evaluation of controlled clinical trials of the effects of feeding donor milk. It is therefore important to proceed to ask what is known of the effects, short and long term, of feeding human milk to preterm babies. Three major areas will be considered: (1) growth and psychomotor development; (2) immunology; and (3) inductive influences.

Growth and Psychomotor Development

Effects on Early Growth

As it has been mentioned earlier, doubts have been repeatedly expressed that growth rates of human milk-fed preterm babies born early in the third trimester are less than adequate ("adequate" usually referring to the rate of intra-uterine growth which would be expected in the normally growing fetus, a widely adopted though by no means proven optimum reference standard of growth for preterm babies). The contemporary rebirth of this concern came in a paper by Davies[2] in 1976, and since this time several other studies have confirmed beyond much doubt that preterm babies fed whatever human milk preparation grow less well in weight, length and head circumference compared with those fed milk formula — both conventional and special low birth-weight formulae.[31–33] A good illustration of this has been provided by Lucas showing that a 1.2 kg baby fed donor human milk would take three weeks longer to reach 2 kg in weight than a baby fed a special preterm weight formula (Figure 1).[33]

One explanation for this slower growth, proposed originally by Gordon and Levine[5] and Powers in America,[6] and resurrected again in the 1970s by Davies[2] and Fomon,[1] is that human milk has insufficient protein to satisfy the avid growth and metabolic needs of prematurely born babies. The amount of nitrogen needed to be retained by the growing fetus at an equivalent developmental age just cannot be provided by mature expressed human milk fed at conventional volumes. The protein concentration of new tissues in preterm babies who are fed human milk is about 30% less than intra-uterine accretion rates.[34] Decreased mineral (calcium and phosphate) bone content is also more prevalent because of an inadequate supply of these minerals: corresponding accretion rates for calcium and phosphorus correspond to only 20% and 30% respectively those in uterus.[35] Critical though protein and mineral insufficiencies might be in limiting growth of preterm infants, another important constituent, largely overlooked in earlier studies, is now considered to be of paramount importance, namely the variable and often remarkably low fat (energy) content of donor human milk which has been discussed earlier. The importance of protein and energy deficiencies as major growth restricting influences can be further deduced from studies where donor human milk enriched with protein, fat and carbohydrate, whether of human or bovine origin, has led to better growth.[36–39]

Figure 1. Weight Gain Curves of Two Preterm Infants Weighing about 1.2 kg at Birth Who Were Fed Respectively a Preterm Formula (PTF) and Banked Breast Milk (BBM).

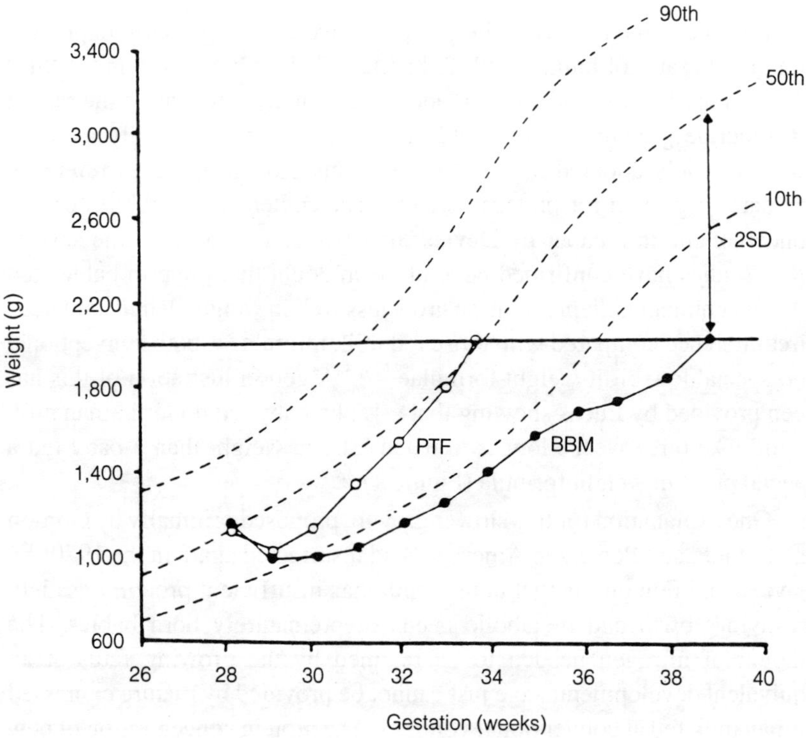

Source: Taken from Lucas, *et al.*[33]

Growth of preterm babies who are fed their own mothers' milk has only recently been investigated.[33,40–42] Lucas[33] reported a small number of preterm babies fed human milk of which at least 95% was from their own mother. There was less weight gain and a lower rate of length and head circumference growth than in those fed a special preterm formula. In contrast to these findings are balance studies showing changes in body composition which, other than for calcium and phosphate where bone rarefaction indicated an insufficient deposition of these minerals, was very similar to the fetus at a comparable developmental age.[43] The fact remains that however motivated are mothers giving birth prematurely, they are usually unable to produce an adequate volume of preterm milk: at most this will amount to only about one-third of their baby's milk requirement.[44] It is for this reason that preterm milk has almost always to be complemented by a "backup diet" of other human milk, milk formula or fortified low birth-weight formula. This necessity further bedevils evaluating the outcome of human milk feeding.

Consequences of Slow Early Growth

Are preterm babies fed human milk who take several weeks to resume growth at an equivalent intra-uterine rate (and who, it is therefore implied, are being undernourished) disadvantaged? In the short term, these young infants have not been shown to be at increased risk of illness: neither should they necessarily have to remain longer in hospital before being discharged home since weight is not the sole determinant for home discharge.[45] That their skeleton may be less than optimally mineralized is beyond dispute but whether this is harmful has yet to be demonstrated.

In the very difficult issue of the long-term effects of poor early growth in preterm babies on later growth and neuro-developmental behaviour, there has been too much uncritical interpolation in the past from studies in small experimental animals where definite permanent and irrecoverable damage in the long term have been shown to follow less than adequate early nutrition. So often the time scale has been out of all proportion and not taken into sufficient account have been the differing developmental stages when inadequate nutrition has been imposed.

Later neuro-developmental status and cognitive function are affected by so many factors — biological, social and environmental — and our current available tools are really very blunt and too imprecise to be able to define significant differences in thought, behaviour, adaptability and reasoning (i.e. intelligence) which might be attributed to early nutritional influences. Notwithstanding these (personal) reservations, such anxieties about long-term influences of less than adequate early nutrition have, without a doubt, had a considerable influence on research and clinical practice directed towards improving nutrition of preterm babies and they cannot be ignored. What have so far been lacking are well-planned long-term studies using sufficient numbers and being able to control as far as possible for the many social and biological variables that also influence intelligence. Encouragingly this hiatus is now being made up through a large British multicentre study coordinated by Lucas and based at the Dunn Nutritional Unit in Cambridge, in which clinical and neuro-developmental outcome in nearly 1,000 babies allocated at random to donor human milk, a preterm approved formula, fortified human milk or standard formula, all given either as a sole feed or supplementary to mothers own milk, is being investigated.[33]

Admitting to these methodological difficulties, what can we deduce so far about these long-term effects?

Physical size Published findings are at variance with each other. Some show a recoverable early growth deficit,[46] others a permanent deficit in size as a consequence of an early period of poor growth.[47] However, I believe much of this divergence of opinion to be due chiefly to differences in experimental approach and an over reliance on *absolute size* as a measure of later adequate growth instead of concentrating attention more on measures of *growth performance*. It is after all impossible to know what should be the true potential for the absolute size of any baby. To illustrate this with one example, preterm births are not equally distributed between social classes, there being an over-representation in lower socio-income groups. Because of a downward gradient in parental size accompanying falling social class, it should not come as too unexpected a finding that a sizeable number of preterm babies will also attain smaller than average size. The effectiveness of attempts to recover the early growth deficit cannot be judged by the sole consideration of absolute size. If attention is focused more on growth performance, such as relating the amount of insufficient early growth to later "catch-up," much of this source of variation should be removed. Using this approach, there is evidence that "catch-up" weight gain is in fact not adversely affected by a period of insufficient early growth[48] in preterm babies. Further work is needed using this model.

Neuro-psychological function The basis of this concern is the slower rate of early head growth that has been described.[2,33] But so many are the genetic and environmental (including not only nutrition and environmental stimulation but also hypoxic influences during the perinatal period) influences on cognitive development that any categoric statement on later psychomotor function related simply to less than adequate nutrition is very difficult to make. Is it really conceivable that a few weeks of less than adequate nutrition during a brain growth spurt lasting at least four years[49] will be to the detriment of both physical growth and neuro-psychological development, as has been implied?[50] After all, many long-term follow-up studies in preterm infants surviving neonatal intensive care point to an excellent outcome in those not developing major neuro-developmental handicap. Early growth has not been accurately documented in most of these studies but periods of poor early growth must have been experienced in many babies since they were born at a time of popularity for feeding human milk. Another reason that I have for questioning a measurable likelihood of long-term detrimental consequences of a few weeks' poor early growth comes from the follow-up of "light-for-dates" babies who would have suffered intra-uterine growth retardation at a developmental stage similar to that of many preterm babies who are growing slowly after birth. For those who do not experience intra-partum asphyxia, the long-term neuro-psychological outlook is excellent, no different from that of normally grown babies born at term.[51]

My innate optimism (without, I have to admit, any scientific basis!) has been slightly eroded recently in reading some early interim findings of the British multicentre study.[33] Babies fed bank human milk have apparently been found significantly shorter at 18 months than those who were fed a special low birth-weight formula. At 9 and 18 months, these babies fed milk formula also showed "significant advantages" in mental and motor function, implying a major consequence to the 20% less brain growth (implied from head circumference differences) during the neonatal period. Is this really conceivable? For reasons previously discussed, I feel uncomfortable about such interim conclusions and await the completed studies with much anticipation.

One important concept relating to brain growth and neuro-psychological outcome has yet to be seriously entertained in the international literature, notably the effects on brain composition of early nutrient intake. Structural (membrane) lipids are made up of esterified phospholipids in which long-chain polyunsaturated fatty acids derived from 18:2w6 and 18:3w3 by elongation-desaturation are principal substrates. During the last trimester of human development, these fatty acids accrue in fetal tissues, especially the brain, with the placenta playing a major role in this synthetic process.[52] The fatty acid composition of human milk seems better suited to make up for the absent placental metabolic processes, and dietary nucleotides in human milk also have the role to facilitate desaturation and elongation of essential fatty acids.[53] Currently available milk formulae do not provide significant amounts of the longer-chain polyunsaturated homologues of 18:2w6 or 18:3w3.[53] Some evidence does exist for an influence on red cell membrane composition from fatty acids in milk[54] with red cell membranes of preterm babies fed human milk having a very different total lipid and fatty acid composition from those fed adapted formulae.[53] We might therefore infer that just as adipose tissue reflects triglyceride composition of the diet so also will some biomembranes. But how do brain cell biomembranes compare in their dietary influences with red cell membranes? How fixed is brain composition? One study, using the thermodynamic characteristics of acetylcholine esterase as a physiological marker, has shown this to be different in erythrocytes from infants fed breast milk compared with butter fat formula.[55] How might this relate to later cognitive development if neural cells are similarly involved? These are important issues that have to be considered alongside simple changes in the gross external physical dimensions of the brain.

Immunological Considerations

Growth and long-term neuro-developmental outcome should not be the sole yardstick to judge the merits of feeding human milk to preterm babies. The "umbrella" of immunological protection, the safety function that permits growth to take place at all, has to be taken into consideration.

Protection against Infection

Antimicrobial substances Human milk contains many antimicrobial substances which have the potential to prevent or modify enteric disease and, also possible, some respiratory tract infections. These substances bridge the immunological gap until the new-born is able to mount its own protection against microbial pathogens. Of particular importance are the milk cells (macrophages, leucocytes and lymphocytes), antibodies (predominantly SIgA), and miscellaneous non-antibody antimicrobial factors (e.g. complement components, lysozyme, nutrient binders such as lactoferrin and vitamin-binding proteins, bifido-bacterium promoting growth factor, low buffering capacity of milk due to low protein and phosphate, volatile fatty acids, lactoperoxidase, etc.).[56] Human milk entering the stomach of preterm babies has also been shown to enhance acid secretion, thus adding further protection from milk-contained bacteria.[57] This umbrella of potential protection, often dependent on complex interactions between the various components, is essential for growth and development to proceed harmoniously. The *in vitro* activity of these antimicrobial substances, which are of especially high concentration in colostrum and early milk, in suppressing bacterial growth is without doubt. That they are important *in vivo* is attested by the many epidemiological studies showing a lower incidence of bacterial and viral gut infections in breast-fed compared with formula-fed babies. They are also probably important for protecting the lactating breast which is especially vulnerable to infection.

Nagging reservations: the need to heat donor milk Unfortunately, the immunological rationale for feeding human milk to preterm babies is not as straightforward as it might initially seem because of the effects of temperature prior to its administration. Milk which is naturally suckled from the breast contains large numbers of bacteria,[26,58] with counts often as high as 10^{10} colony forming units (CFU)/ml. The predominant organisms are normal skin flora (St. epidermidis, Str. viridans) but potential pathogens are also found. Donor milk has a similar flora arising from inadequately sterilized equipment, collecting utensils and nosocomial contamination, and so on. Ingesting milk containing these micro-organisms seems not to provide any real hazard to the healthy term baby, presumably because of specific prenatally acquired antibody protection from the mother aided by the many substances in milk and its own gastric acid. But for the gestationally immature infant who is deprived of much transplacental antibody and with an immune system less able to cope with potentially hostile micro-organisms, contamination of donor milk is widely presumed to be a risk factor for neonatal infection even though preterm infants might be able to absorb IgA and even IgG from their own mothers' milk.[59]

Even with careful collection procedures which give meticulous attention to washing and sterilizing equipment, it is inevitable that micro-organisms will enter the milk[58,60] with median counts difficult to be kept below 10^3 CFU/ml. It is this presence of micro-organisms, harmless commensals as well as potential pathogens, that underlies the widespread practice of pasteurizing donor milk (other than that provided by the baby's own mother which is usually given "raw") before feeding to babies in order to make it microbiologically "safe." Human milk can also be an important vector for transmission of viruses within specific milk cells. Recent studies drawing attention to transmission of Hepatitis B surface antigen, Cytomegalovirus and now Human Immunodeficiency Virus (HIV)[61] (which are all destroyed by careful pasteurization) have further vindicated this practice although it remains to be conclusively shown that such transmission via milk actually causes disease or carrier states in the new-born.

It is unfortunate therefore that pasteurizing human milk destroys many of the substances with powerful antimicrobial properties, humoral and cellular, with the harm directly related to the temperature to which the milk is subjected (Table 3).[62–65] It also appears unlikely that any method of collecting human milk will allow the baby to receive immunologically functional cells since these are easily damaged by any heat and they adhere to the walls of the collecting and feeding bottles.[64] Rendering human milk immunologically impotent by high temperatures has led some paediatricians to recommend feeding babies donor human milk which has not been heated, and it is claimed without apparent ill effect. Some reports have been made of outbreaks of infection on Neonatal Units traced to contaminated banked breast milk but as a general statement, there is surprisingly little evidence linking infection in babies to feeding unheated milk. Indeed, the converse might equally as well apply that destruction of protective substances reduces the ability of heated human milk to resist bacterial growth. There are no microbiologically agreed criteria for feeding milk in a raw state, although some have been proposed,[58] but by many the practice is considered dangerous in view of infection risks.

Table 3. The Percentage Survival of Some Protective Antimicrobial Factors in Human Milk after Heat Treatment at Different Temperatures for Different Periods of Time.[62–65]

Antimicrobial factor	Temperatures in C° and time of exposure to heat in minutes					
	56°×30′	62.5°×30′	70°×15′	73°×30′	100°×3′	100°×15′
Immunoglobulin A	96	67–100	48	0	0	0
Immunoglobulin M	100	0				
Lysozyme		64–100	65	2	0	3
Lactoferrin		40–100	5	1		0
Vitamin B_{12} binding capacity		52	33			43
Folic acid binding capacity		90	65			7

The perennial question therefore is whether the immunological and nutritional benefits of feeding unheated donor milk outweigh the potential hazards of exposing babies to risks of illness from milk which is likely to be contaminated with bacteria or viruses? The answer is not known but social and environmental factors play a decisive role in the eventual decision. In the developing world, where risks of perinatal nosocomial infection are very high and with formula feeding a major risk factor for enteric disease, the strongest possible case exists to give donor milk (which in most instances will be mother's own milk) unheated, providing that care is taken to express milk under the best possible hygienic conditions. Advantages conferred by feeding milk containing virtually unaltered immunological substances will far outweigh the potential disadvantages of causing infection. An important study undertaken in New Delhi by Narayanan and her colleagues in 1984 convincingly showed that feeding unheated expressed donor breast milk to low birth-weight infants especially at risk of infection significantly diminished the incidence of systemic neonatal sepsis.[66] Especially interesting was that of 454 samples of milk taken immediately before feeding, 22% grew non-pathogenic organisms and 13% potential pathogens (E. Coli, Klebsiella, St. Aureus): but in none of the infants who were fed milk containing these potential pathogens could these be implicated in causing infection. Similar experiences have been recently reported by Olowe from Nigeria where 30% of milk samples fed to babies on a neonatal unit contained potentially pathogenic organisms yet no disease was attributable to this milk. Continued use of this unscreened expressed breast milk furthermore dramatically reduced the incidence of nosocomial gastroenteritis.[60]

In more developed parts of the world where high overall standards of perinatal care lead to a low incidence of infection in new-born nurseries, and where formula feeding is associated with minimal risk, the anti-infective advantages of feeding raw milk are more difficult to ascertain. In this environment, vividly contrasting with that in so many developing countries, there is as yet no convincing evidence for breast milk conferring additional advantage against infections: risks of causing nosocomial infection from feeding unheated human milk are seen by many to outweigh theoretical advantages. But even this issue is not without its controversy. Over the years, several correspondents to medical journals have admitted that their practice has been not to heat milk and that this has not caused any noticeable increase in infection rates. This applies especially in

Sweden where non-pasteurized milk has been given for many years. Maybe therefore the theoretical dangers are being exaggerated. “Safe” levels of bacterial contamination have not been established although normal nursing infants have been shown to digest between 10^2 to 10^6 CFU/ml during a feed with no harmful consequence.[58]

This controversy will be resolved only through carefully controlled clinical trials but regrettably the impetus for such studies seems now to have been removed in favour of nutritional considerations and the fear of transmitting certain viruses, especially Cytomegalovirus, HIV and Hepatitis B. So far, cases of illness have only rarely been linked to directly suckled milk containing these viruses — perhaps because of the mitigating influences of transplacental protective substances and in the breast milk. Notwithstanding, I am sure that few milk banks in developed countries would now risk giving unheated milk. Holder pasteurization (62˚C for 30 minutes), a process derived from the method employed to destroy M. Tuberculosis in bovine milk and empirically transcribed to human milk, is the method most widely recommended to achieve a satisfactory reduction in the number of contained micro-organisms,[3] thereby rendering the milk safe for feeding, and preserving as far as possible its antimicrobial properties. 99% of bacterial contaminants will be destroyed providing the CF counts are $< 10^7$ CFU/ml at the outset. Human milk can be effectively pasteurized using lower temperatures for a shorter time (e.g. 56˚C for 15 minutes; 62.5˚C for 5 minutes), at the same time preserving substantially more of its antimicrobial properties,[67] but this approach is not widely adopted.

Prevention of Necrotizing Enterocolitis

Part of the price which is currently being paid for the increased survival of very small preterm babies appear in many neonatal units to be an increase in the incidence of necrotizing enterocolitis (NEC). In an experimental rat animal model, fresh milk of the same species has been shown to protect against this serious condition,[68,69] the explanation proposed being that the immune substances in milk, particularly secretary IgA cells, suppress the colonization of the bowel with potential pathogenic organisms (especially perhaps clostridia, Klebsiella) which seem an essential prerequisite for the condition in babies where there has been some intestine ischaemia. Mizrahi in 1965[70] was the first to suggest that breast milk protected against NEC and in 1987 a report by the American Academy of Pediatrics Committee on Nutrition stated: "This frequently fatal condition is rare in low birth-weight, breast-fed neonates."[71] Careful examination of available data does not however substantiate these views,[72–74] even when fresh as opposed to pasteurized whole milk is given. It might of course be that the discrepancy between the convincing animal model and the real life human situation is due to the loss of immune substances and cells during the process of the preparation (heat), storage (cold) and administration of the milk. There is yet no convincing evidence to support the proposition that feeding human milk to preterm babies lessens the risks of NEC. Recently however an oral immunoglobulin supplement (73% IgA, 26% IgG) has been shown to prevent NEC in babies weighing < 2,000 g at birth, an effect speculated to be due to the combining of immunoglobulin with bacterial antigen to prevent bowel wall adherence of bacteria. This finding adds some theoretical basis for the protective value of human milk: failure to show this *in practice* might simply reflect the much lower concentration of SIgA in human milk than in the oral immunoglobulin supplement.

Protection against Protein Antigen-related Disorders

β-lactoglobulin, the major whey protein in cow's milk, is absorbed in large amounts as antigenically intact protein by preterm babies fed milk formulae.[75] (Indeed, many of the "humanized" milks now available will, due to higher whey/casein ratios, make available much more β-lactoglobulin than in less modified formulae.) The more gestationally immature the baby the greater the gut permeability. For example, preterm babies less than 33 weeks' gestation have absorption rates up to 100-fold greater than those in term infants.[75] Intact β-lactoglobulin is of no nutritional value to the baby but theoretically it might initiate an immune response with potentially worrying consequences for the development of later allergic disease. Early latent anaphylactic sensitation of blood basophils has been described in association with cow's milk protein feeding[76] but as yet there is no evidence that atopic disease and other allergies are any more common in preterm than in term babies whatever the mode of feeding. Notwithstanding, there should always be awareness of these possibilities whenever the choice of food is considered. Human milk, though containing some foreign protein from the mother,[77] should at least in theory offer maximum protection against this category of illness. Further long-term studies are awaited to explore the possible long-term consequences of early foreign protein ingress.

Inductive Properties of Human Milk

In addition to nutrient and immunological constituents, a third group of components in human milk which are increasingly becoming the source of much interest are growth modulators and other physiological substances, such as enzymes and hormones.[78] Growth modulators are mainly low molecular weight peptides found in milk of many species and appear to be principally concerned with improving early growth and differentiation of the gastrointestinal mucosa to aid its functional adaptation to the demands of enteral nutrition. These collectively can be termed the inductive properties of milk. Examples of such growth factors include taurine, ethanolamine, phospho-ethanolamine, epidermal growth factor, nerve growth factor.[78] Widdowson, in a seminal early investigation, studied pigs and rabbits who had been naturally suckled compared with those starved for 24 hours.[79] The enteric mucosa was 75% heavier and contained 50% more DNA in those who suckled. The presence of these growth modulator substances which are especially rich in colostrum and early milk perhaps explains why, compared with formula-fed preterm babies, human milk feeding causes less vomiting and gastric stasis.

Some growth factors might also have a metabolic role on target organs outside the gastrointestinal tract after being absorbed into the circulation. For example taurine, as a free amino acid, has its greatest concentration in the fetal brain in the second trimester.[78] Might it be important for brain maturation? This possibility has led to its inclusion in some of the new preterm formulae. Of the sixty or so enzymes in human milk so far defined, little is known of their *in vivo* activities other than bile salt-stimulated lipase which has a well-defined role in helping triglyceride digestion, making up for immature pancreatic function.[80] Denaturation of this enzyme by heat has been held accountable for the slower weight gain in pasteurized milk-fed babies.[26] Might such treatment affect other enzymes? Certainly dietary nucleotides, part of the non-protein nitrogen component have been shown to help the *in vivo* desaturation and elongation of fatty acids to form long-chain polyunsaturated fatty acids needed for membrane synthesis.[53]

Preterm babies not fed human milk would be deprived of these inductive properties. So far this deprivation has not been linked with any measurable ill effects. Their definition has however served to emphasize once again the biological complexity of human milk with its immune substances, growth modulators, enzymes and hormones facilitating the best possible assimilation of its nutrients.

Conclusion

Finkelstein[4] would be intrigued to discover sixty years further on that the doubts and anxieties which he had raised over the adequacy of breast milk for preterm babies were still being fiercely debated. Barrie, from Charing Cross Hospital, London, has provided an example of strongly held opinion.[81] In a letter to the *Lancet* in 1982, he said that he was not prepared to use donor milk under any circumstances, using the issue of iatrogenic problems associated with giving donor milk as the strongest argument against its use. Lucas' recent findings of significant hyperbilirubinaemia in donor milk-fed babies[82] might be considered an interesting additional potential iatrogenic hazard, though one which with modern methods of treatment should not cause any serious ill effects. Timely though these warning might be, compared with other fearful sources of iatrogenesis in small babies looked after in neonatal intensive care units, these risks are likely to be small, provided of course that due care is taken. Indeed, it is salutary to recall that the most serious iatrogenic problems associated with infant feeding practices in recent years were those of hypernatraemia and hypocalcaemia from high solute artificial milk feeding in the 1960s and early 1970s.

I would finally like to offer my views on the suitability of human milk for prematurely born babies bringing together the various arguments I have previously put forward.

First, mothers giving birth prematurely should be given every encouragement to express and feed their own milk in the freshest possible condition to their baby. I contend there is no need to submit this milk to bacterial screening nor to heat this milk, providing it is collected in such a way as to minimize bacterial contamination, kept carefully in a refrigerator at 4°C (with minimal opening and closing of the door to reduce swings in temperature) and given within about 24 to 48 hours. (Human milk once collected is remarkably resistant to bacterial growth for at least 5 days.)

Beyond this time, Holder pasteurization will be needed. Even if the nutritional and immunological arguments for feeding this preterm milk are not particularly strong, expressing her own milk will give the mother something positive to do at a time when she feels helpless yet is eager to do something to help her baby. If the mother's milk cannot be used within about 48 hours, the milk should be pasteurized and then kept at –20°C until required. This will preserve as far as possible the antimicrobial substances (except for the cells) so that when the milk is later thawed and administered, some potential benefits will still be conferred. If as is likely this preterm milk is not available in adequate amounts, then a complementary "backup" feed of human milk or conventionally used milk formula will also need to be given.

Second, preterm babies born in *less affluent countries* and who are at particular risk of gastrointestinal infection must be given their own mothers milk complemented wherever possible by expressed milk from other mothers in hospital (under close supervision to minimize contamination). There can be no denying the vital importance of human milk given in the freshest possible condition to these babies.

Third, for preterm babies born in *developed regions* of the world whose mothers do not wish to express their own milk and where, because of hygienic perinatal practices, the risks of infection are low, the decision is less simple. Most opinion in countries where milk banking practices have been part of the scene for many years and where there has been in the recent decade a remarkable resurgence in breast-feeding, would continue to encourage its use despite the many reservations that have been voiced. Old customs die hard and I also tend to adhere to this view. A report, "The Collection and Storage of Human Milk,"[56] commissioned by the Department of Health and Social Security in Britain in 1981, reflects this confidence, and offers very comprehensive practical guidelines for the setting up and organization of milk banking practices, including the best methods for milk collection and donor selection to avoid transmission of organisms, nutritional state, drugs, to give the best possible food.

Lacto-engineering, the process by which nutrient composition of donor milk is improved by fortifying with specific nutrients, fat, protein and minerals, to give an enriched human milk formula, can be included in this recommendation.[83] Fortifying human milk with calcium and phosphate undoubtedly improves mineral balance but accretion still falls below estimated intra-uterine rates. Growth rates have been shown to benefit.[36]

Lacto-engineering minimizes compositional variability of human milk although the technology and infrastructure demanded by this process are complex and very costly, involving centrifugation, dialysis and freeze drying, demands which are beyond the capabilities of most hospital milk banks. This approach is exciting however since if the method of modifying human milk can be shown to better provide the nutritional and immunological needs of small babies, the impetus to develop the method on a wider scale will be very real. The outcome, both long-term and short-term, of clinical trials using such strategies to improve the nutrient content of human milk formulae are awaited with interest. However, the current realities, disappointingly, are that lacto-engineering research will probably slow down considerably since, with recommendations that all donating mothers should now be screened for HIV and other viruses, such as hepatitis and Cytomegalovirus, the supply of milk will inevitably fall severely.[84] The future may therefore be concerned more with the fortification of mother's own milk with cow's milk ingredients (protein and minerals) and medium-chain triglycerides.

It does however appear to me that human milk feeding for preterm babies is now gradually falling into disrepute in many modern neonatal units the world over since clear advantages have not been demonstrated over new sophisticated formulae. However, I still have a nagging doubt that with so much left to learn about its many nutritional, immunological and inductive properties, it would be best not to dispense too hastily with human milk. Is it not important to demonstrate that artificial milk formulae, made up chiefly from dairy products, vegetable fats and proteins fortified with vitamins and iron, achieve better short and long-term results for preterm babies than does donor human milk, in spite of its nutritional imperfections? Hopefully some of these questions will be answered by the ongoing British Multicentre Study.[33] What also of the current interest in the early metabolic programming (long-term effects of an environmental stimulus at sensitive points in metabolic development) by human milk on disease in later life, especially the premature onset of ischaemic heart disease and hypertension.[85] There is no reason why arguments applied to term babies in relation to early fat, cholesterol and sodium intake should not be equally applicable to babies born before term. Figure 2 summarizes the dilemma, but offers no easy solution.

Fourth, relevance for Hong Kong. Should we be encouraging the collection and use of human milk for preterm babies in Hong Kong where

Figure 2. The Dilemma of Human Milk Feeding for Preterm Babies.

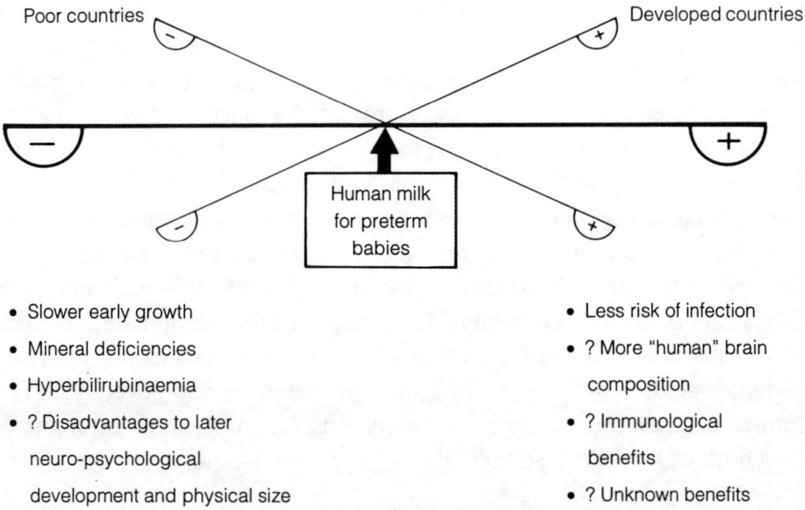

the incidence of breast-feeding is currently extremely low? Whatever the ideals, realities are that we cannot isolate the arguments for breast-feeding from prevailing socio-economic conditions and attitudes. We should all be working towards improving the climate of opinion which would favour breast-feeding, since this after all is what Nature has intended for the human infant, but to do this without regard to complex social predicaments is to sometimes weaken the case and to render improvement difficult. The same argument will also apply to the feeding of human milk to preterm babies, and I make the admission as one heavily committed to the ideals and practice of feeding human milk to preterm babies when I was working in the United Kingdom in the 1970s.

If there is sufficient motivation and expertise available, mothers should be encouraged to collect their own milk and feed it to their babies, but with the full realization that the organization involved in hospital milk banking practices, however simple, is extremely demanding, requiring a real commitment on the part of mothers, medical and nursing staff. There needs to be a system of delivery of milk within and to the hospital; microbiological systems for safety purposes and even some form of nutritional quality control for fat content. Where a framework exists, it is sensible to continue with it. If such an infrastructure does not exist however, then the cost and management skills which are demanded (at a time when so many anxieties are being expressed over the suitability of donor human milk for preterm babies and where the formula alternatives are undoubtedly capable of providing adequate nutrients to satisfy as well as possible growth and other requirements), in my opinion, militate against the setting up of milk banks. It would be prudent instead to await the findings of further research into the merits of donor milk before embarking on such a labour-intensive programme.

I will leave the last words to Dr. F. Ford, a Glasgow paediatrician, who in 1949 made a statement as apposite now as when it was written forty years ago:

> When breast milk can be obtained from a milk bank it is expensive in money and when the bank is part of a hospital's activity it is expensive in nurses' time. It is, therefore, essential to find out if breast milk is really so advantageous as to justify the financial outlay and the use of valuable nursing hours in collecting and processing it.[86]

These words provide a salutary reminder of how little we have achieved and how much needs to be done to establish the true value of human milk for preterm babies.

Acknowledgements

I thank Miss Juliet Lee for her time and infinite patience in preparing this manuscript.

References

1. Fomon, S. J., Ziegler, E. E., and Vazquez, H. D. Human Milk and the Small Premature Infant. *Am J Dis Child*, 1977; 131:463–67.
2. Davies, D. P. Adequacy of Expressed Breast Milk for Early Growth of Preterm Infants. *Arch Dis Child*, 1977; 52:296–301.
3. Baum, J. D. The Effects of Pasteurization on Immune Factors in Human Milk. In Visser, H. K., ed., *Nutrition and Metabolism of the Fetus and Infant*. Boston: Nijhoff, 1979; 173–83.
4. Finkelstein, H. *Lehrbuch der Sauglingskrankheiten*. Berlin: Springer, 1912. Referred to by Powers (1948) (see Reference 6).
5. Gordon, H. H., Levine, S. Z., and McNamara, H. Feeding of Premature Infants: A Comparison of Human and Cow's Milk. *Am J Dis Child*, 1947; 73:442–52.

6. Powers, G. F. Some Observations on the Feeding of Premature Infants Based on 20 Years' Experience at the New Haven Hospital. *Pediatrics*, 1947; 1: 145–58.
7. Department of Health and Social Security. The Composition of Mature Human Milk. *Reports on Health and Social Subjects*, No. 12. London: HMSO, 1977.
8. Carroll, L., Conlan, D., and Davies, D. P. Fat Content of Bank Human Milk. *Arch Dis Child*, 1980; 55:969.
9. Gibbs, J. H., Fisher, C., Bhattacharya, S., *et al.* Drip Breast Milk: Its Composition, Collection and Pasteurization. *Early Hum Dev*, 1977; 1:227–45.
10. Lucas, A., Gibbs, J.A.H., and Baum, J. D. The Biology of Human Drip Breast Milk. *Early Hum Dev*, 1978; 2:351–59.
11. Stocks, R., Davies, D. P., Carroll, L., *et al.* A Simple Method to Improve the Energy Value of Bank Human Milk. *Early Hum Dev*, 1983; 8:175–78.
12. Finley, D.A.C., and Lonnerdal, B. Fatty Acid Composition of Breast Milk from Vegetarian and Non-vegetarian Lactating Women. In Schaub, J., ed., *Composition and Physiological Properties of Human Milk.* Amsterdam: Elsevier Science Publishers, Biomedical Division, 1985; 203–12.
13. Atkinson, S. A., Bryan, M. H., and Anderson, G. H. Human Milk: Difference in Nitrogen Concentration in Milk from Mothers of Term and Premature Infants. *J Pediatr*, 1978; 93:67–69.
14. Atkinson, S. A., Anderson, G. H., and Bryan, M. H. Human Milk: Comparison of the Nitrogen Composition in Milk from Mothers or Premature and Full-term Infants. *Am J Clin Nutr*, 1980; 33:811–15.
15. Atkinson, S. A., Radde, I. C., Chance, G. W., *et al.* Macromineral Content of Milk Obtained during Early Lactation from Mothers of Premature Infants. *Early Hum Dev*, 1980; 4:5–14.
16. Gross, S. J., David, R. J., Burman, L., *et al.* Nutritional Composition of Milk Produced by Mothers Delivering Preterm. *J Pediatr*, 1980; 96:641–44.
17. Koo, W.W.K., and Gupta, J. M. Breast Milk Sodium. *Arch Dis Child*, 1982; 57:500–2.
18. Lemons, J. A., Moye, L., Hall, D., *et al.* Differences in the Composition of Preterm and Term Milk during Early Lactation. *Pediatr Res*, 1982; 16:113–17.
19. Schanler, R. J., and Oh, W. Composition of Breast Milk Obtained from Mothers of Premature Infants as Compared to Breast Milk Obtained from Donors. *J Pediatr*, 1980; 96:679–81.
20. Atkinson, S. A., Anderson, G. H., and Bryan, M. H. Energy Content of Human Milk during Early Lactation from Mothers Giving Birth Prematurely. *Am J Clin Nutr*, 1979; 32:78.
21. Lucas, A., Suzuki, S., and Coombs, R.R.A. IgA and Preterm Milk. *Lancet*, 1982; 1:1,242–43.
22. Gross, S. J., Buckley, R. H., Wakil, S. S., *et al.* Elevated IgA Concentration

in Milk Provided by Mothers Delivered of Preterm Infants. *J Pediatr*, 1981; 99:389–93.

23. Hamosh, M., Bitman, C. S., *et al.* Lipid Composition of Preterm Human Milk and Its Digestion by the Infant. In Schaub, J., ed., *Composition and Physiological Properties of Human Milk.* Amsterdam: Elsevier Science Publishers, Biomedical Division, 1985; 153–62.
24. Murphy, J. F., Neals, M. L., and Matthews, N. Antimicrobial Properties of Preterm Breast Milk Cells. *Arch Dis Child*, 1983; 58:198–200.
25. Goldham, A. S., Garza, C., Nichols, B. L., *et al.* Effects of Prematurity on the Immunological System in Human Milk. *J Pediatr*, 1982; 101:901–10.
26. Williamson, S., Finucane, E., Ellis, H., *et al.* Effect of Heat Treatment of Human Milk on Absorption of Nitrogen, Fat, Sodium, Calcium and Phosphorus by Preterm Infants. *Arch Dis Child*, 1978; 53:555–63.
27. Hernell, O., and Blackberg, L. Lipolysis in Human Milk: Causes and Consequences. In Schaub, J., ed., *Composition and Physiological Properties of Human Milk.* Amsterdam: Elsevier Science Publishers, Biomedical Division, 1985; 115–28.
28. Paxson, C. L., Cress, C. C. Survival of Human Milk Leukocytes. *J Pediatr*, 1979; 94:61–68.
29. Brook, O. G., and Barley, J. Loss of Energy during Continuous Infusions of Breast Milk. *Arch Dis Child*, 1978; 53:344–45.
30. Stocks, R., Davies, D. P., Allen, F., *et al.* Loss of Breast Milk Nutrients during Tude Feeding. *Arch Dis Child*, 1985; 60:164–67.
31. Tudehope, D. I., Mitchell, F., and Cowley, D. M. A Comparative Study of a Premature Infant Formula and Preterm Breast Milk for Low Birthweight Infants. *Aust Paediatr J*, 1986; 22:199–205.
32. Brooke, O. G., Onuboju, O., Heath, R., *et al.* Human Milk and Preterm Formula Compared for Effects on Growth and Metabolism. *Arch Dis Child*, 1987; 62:917–23.
33. Lucas, A., Gore, S. M., Cole, T. J., *et al.* A Multicentre Trial on the Feeding of Low Birthweight Infants: Effects of Diet on Early Growth. *Arch Dis Child*, 1984; 59:702–30.
34. Roberts, S. B., and Lucas, A. The Effects of Two Extremes of Dietary Intake on Protein Accretion in Preterm Infants. *Early Hum Dev*, 1985; 12:301–7.
35. Santerre, J., and Salle, B. Calcium and Phosphorus Economy of the Preterm Infants and Its Interaction with Vitamin D and Its Metabolites. *Acta Paed Scand* (Suppl.), 1982; 296:85–92.
36. Modanlou, H. D., Lim, M. O., Hasen, J. W., *et al.* Growth, Biochemical Status and Mineral Metabolism in Very-low-birth-weight Infants Receiving Fortified Preterm Human Milk. *J Pediatr Gastroenterol Nutr*, 1986; 5:762–67.
37. Spencer, S. A., Stammers, J. P., and Hull, D. Evaluation of a Special Low

Birth-weight Formula, with and without the Use of Medium Chain Triglyceride. *Early Hum Dev*, 1986; 13:87–95.
38. Schanler, R. J., Garza, C., and Nichols, B. L. Fortified Mother's Milk for Very-low-birth-weight Infants: Results of Growth and Nutrient Balance Studies. *J Pediatr*, 1985; 107:437–45.
39. Bustamante, S. A., Fiello, A., and Pollack, P. F. Growth of Premature Infants Fed Formulas with 10%, 30%, or 50% Medium-chain Triglycerides. *Am J Dis Child*, 1987; 141:516–19.
40. Atkinson, S. A., Radde, I. C., and Anderson, G. H. Macromineral Balances in Premature Infants Fed Their Own Mothers' Milk or Formula. *J Pediatr*, 1983; 102:99–106.
41. Chessex, P., Reichman, B., Verellen, G., *et al.* Human Milk Stimulates the Quality of Fetal Growth in Premature Infants. *Pediatr Res*, 1984; 4:159 (A).
42. Gross, S. J. Growth and Biomedical Response of Preterm Infants Formula. *N Engl J Med*, 1982; 308:237–41.
43. Reichman, B., Chessex, P., Verellen, G., *et al.* Dietary Composition and Macronutrient Storage in Preterm Infants. *Pediatrics*, 1983; 72:322–28.
44. Lucas, A. Availability of Preterm Milk. *Lancet*, 1985; 2:891–99.
45. Derbyshire, F., Davies, D. P., and Bacco, A. Discharge of Preterm Babies from Neonatal Units. *BMJ*, 1982; 284:233–34.
46. Fitzharding, P. M. Early Growth and Development in Low Birthweight Infants Following Treatment in an Intensive Care Nursery. *Pediatrics*, 1975; 56: 162–69.
47. Babson, S. G. Growth of Low Birthweight Infants. *J Pediatr*, 1970; 77:11–18.
48. Davies, D. P., and Kennedy, J. D. Insufficient Early Weight Gain in Preterm Babies and Influence on Weight at 12 Months. *Arch Dis Child*, 1985; 60: 718–21.
49. Dobbing, J., and Sands, J. Quantitative Growth and Development of Human Brain. *Arch Dis Child*, 1973; 48:757.
50. Tyson, J., Lasky, R., Mize, C., *et al.* Growth and Development of Infants Less Than 1,500g Fed Bank Human Milk or Premature Formula. *Pediatr Res*, 1981; 15:549.
51. Westwood, M., Kramer, M. S., Munz, D., *et al.* Growth and Development of Full-term Non-asphyxiated Small-for-gestational Age Newborns: Follow-up through Adolescence. *Pediatrics*, 1983; 71:376.
52. Crawford, M., Hassam, A. G., Williams, G., *et al.* Essential Fatty Acids and Fetal Brain Growth. *Lancet*, 1978; 1:452–54.
53. Clandinen, M. T., and Chapell, J. E. Long Chain Polyenoic Fatty Acids in Human Milk: Are They of Benefit to the Newborn. In Schaub, J., ed., *Composition and Physiological Properties of Human Milk.* Amsterdam: Elsevier Science Publishers, Biomedical Division, 1985; 213–24.

54. Delucchi, C., Pita, M. L., Faus, M. J., *et al.* Effects of Dietary Nucleotides on the Fatty Acid Composition of Erythrocyte Membrane Lipids in Term Infants. *J Pediatr Gastroenterol Nutr*, 1987; 6:568–74.
55. Hall, B., Muller, D.P.R., Agget, P. J., *et al.* The Effect of Milk Lipids on the Activity of Acetylcholine Esterase in Red Blood Cells. In Schaub, J., ed., *Composition and Physiological Properties of Human Milk.* Amsterdam: Elsevier Science Publishers, Biomedical Division, 1985; 179–88.
56. Department of Health and Social Security Panel on Child Nutrition. The Collection and Storage of Human Milk. Working Party Report on Human Milk Banks. *Reports on Health and Social Subjects*, No. 22. London: HMSO, 1981.
57. Usowicz, A. G., Dab, S. B., Emery, J. R., *et al.* Does Gastric Acid Protect the Preterm Infant from Bacteria in Unheated Milk. *Early Hum Dev*, 1988; 16: 27–34.
58. Carroll, L., Davies, D. P., Osman, M., *et al.* Bacteriological Criteria for Feeding Raw Breast Milk to Babies on Neonatal Units. *Lancet*, 1979; 2:732–34.
59. Savilahti, E., Jarvenpaa, A. L., and Rahiha, N.C.R. Serum Immunoglobins in Preterm Infants: Comparisons of Human Milk and Formula Feeding. *Pediatrics*, 1983; 72:312–16.
60. Olowe, S. A., Ahmed, I., Lawol, S. F., *et al.* Bacterial Quality of Raw Human Milk: Effect of Storage in a Refrigerator. *Ann Trop Paediatr*, 1987; 7:233–37.
61. Thiry, L., Sprecher-Goldberger, S., Jonckeer, T., *et al.* Isolation of AIDS Virus from Cell Free Breast Milk of Three Healthy Virus Carriers. *Lancet*, 1985; 2:891–92.
62. Evans, T. J., Ryley, H. C., Neale, L. M., *et al.* Effect of Storage and Heat on Antimicrobial Proteins in Human Milk. *Arch Dis Child*, 1978; 53:239–41.
63. Ford, J. E., Law, B. A., Marshall, V.M.E., *et al.* Influence of the Heat Treatment of Human Milk on Some of Its Protective Constituents. *J Pediatr*, 1977; 90:29–35.
64. Leibharber, M., Lewiston, N. J., Asquith, T. T., *et al.* Lymphocytes and Antibody Content of Human Milk after Processing. *J Pediatr*, 1977; 91:897–900.
65. Rapotopoulou-Gigi, M., Marwick, K., and McClelland, D.B.L. Antimicrobial Proteins in Sterilized Human Milk. *BMJ*, 1977; 1:12–14.
66. Narayanan, I., Prakash, K., Bala, S., *et al.* Randomized Controlled Trial of Effect of Raw and Holder Pasteurized Human Milk and of Formula Supplements on Incidence of Neonatal Infection. *Lancet*, 1984; 2:1,111–13.
67. Wills, M. E., Han, V. E., and Harris, D. A. Short Time Low Temperature Pasteurization of Human Milk. *Early Hum Dev*, 1983; 7:71–73.
68. Barlow, B., Santulli, T. V., Heird, W. C., *et al.* An Experimental Study of Acute Neonatal Enterocolitis. *Pediatr Surg*, 1974; 9:587–95.
69. Pitt, J., Barlow, B., Heird, W. C., *et al.* Neonatal Enterocolitis: Possible Pathogenesis. *Pediatr Res*, 1974; 8:384.

70. Mizrahi, A., Barlow, B., Berdon, W., *et al.* Necrotizing Enterocolitis in Premature Infants. *J Pediatr*, 1965; 66:697–99.
71. Committee on Nutrition of the American Academy of Pediatrics. Breast Feeding. *Pediatrics*, 1978; 62:591–601.
72. *Communicable Disease Report*, 82.05.3. London: Public Health Laboratory Service, 1982.
73. Reisner, S. H., and Garty, B. Necrotizing Enterocolitis Despite Breast Feeding. *Lancet*, 1977; 3:507.
74. Stoll, B. J., Kanto, W. P., Glass, R. L., *et al.* Epidemiology of Necrotizing Enterocolitis. *J Pediatr*, 1980; 96:447–57.
75. Robertson, D. M., Panganelli, R., Dinwiddie, R., *et al.* Milk Antigen Absorption in the Preterm and Term Neonates. *Arch Dis Child*, 1982; 57:369–72.
76. Lucas, A., McLaughlan, P., and Coombs, R.R.A. Latent Anaphylactic Sensitization of Infants of Low Birth-weight to Cow's Milk Proteins. *BMJ*, 1984; 289:1,254–56.
77. Evans, R. W., Allardyce, D. M., Fergusson, D. M., *et al.*, Maternal Diet and Infantile Colic in Breast Fed Infants. *Lancet*, 1981; 1:1,340–42.
78. Gaull, G. E., Isaacs, C. E., Wright, C. E., *et al.* Growth Modulators in Human Milk: Implications for Milk Banking. In Williams, A. F., and Baum, J. D., eds., *Human Milk Banking*. Nestle Nutrition; New York: Vevey/Raven Press, 1984; 63–71.
79. Widdowson, E. M., Colombo, V. E., and Artavanis, C. A. Changes in the Organs of Pigs in Response to Feeding for the First 24 Hours after Birth — II. The Digestive Tract. *Biol Neonate*, 1976; 35:131–42.
80. Freed, L. M., York, C. M., Hamosh, P., *et al.* Bile-salt Stimulated Lipase of Human Milk: Characteristics of Enzyme in the Milk of Mothers of Premature and Full Term Infants. *J Pediatr Gastroenterol Nutr*, 1987; 6:598–604.
81. Barrie, H. Human Milk Banks. *Lancet*, 1982; 1:284.
82. Lucas, A., and Barker, B. A. Breast Milk Jaundice in Premature Infants. *Arch Dis Child*, 1986; 61:1,063–67.
83. Gaiza, C., Schanler, R. J., Goldman, A. S., *et al.* Preparation and Evaluation of Fortified Human Milk for Very Low Birth-weight Infants. In Williams, A. F., and Baum, J. D., eds., *Human Milk Banking*. Nestle Nutrition; New York: Vevey/Raven Press, 1984; 101–11.
84. Breast Not Necessarily Best (editorial). *Lancet*, 1988; 1:624–25.
85. Infant Nutrition and Cardiovascular Disease. *Scientific Report No. 8*. Southampton: M.R.C. Environmental Epidemiology Unit, 1987.
86. Ford, F. J. Feeding of Premature Babies. *Lancet*, 1949; 1:987–94

6

"Catch-up" Growth in Deprived Children

The Hong Kong Journal of Paediatrics, 1987; 4:63–65

Summary

Two children, casualties of severe early psycho-social deprivation after being abandoned early in their lives, showed remarkable "catch-up" growth in height when their psychological and social environments improved. Deprived children in special institutions and orphanages should have their physical growth regularly monitored as part of their ongoing assessment in order to provide an objective marker of their progress.

Introduction

Growth failure is a frequent accompaniment of child abuse. A recent study from Sheffield[1] has shown how physical growth performance can provide an important marker of recovery in the follow up of children who have been admitted to hospital suffering proven abuse: better placement resulting in greatest "catch-up" growth. The present two case histories extend this observation into another important aspect of social paediatrics, namely some of the consequences of early socio-cultural deprivation.

Case Histories

Case 1

A girl born illegitimate was abandoned by her mother at nine months. She was made a ward of the Director of Social Welfare after which she was placed in three residential homes one after another. She was found unable to cope with the environment, demonstrating marked retardation in motor, language and social development, severe behavioural problems and emotionally unstable. Psychological assessment identified her as moderate grade mentally handicapped and at the age of three years, she was placed in a residential preschool centre for mentally handicapped children. Gradually she became more secure and emotionally stable and her behaviour and educational abilities showed marked improvement. At the age of six years, she was able to attend a kindergarten for normal children with above average academic achievement. A year later, she left the centre to live with adoptive parents overseas. Her growth in height since entering the school is shown in Figure 1 (children in the centre have their height measured every six months). This demonstrates remarkable "catch-up."

Case 2

A boy was abandoned in hospital when a few weeks old. He was taken into a children's service centre where he developed psychological emotional problems. Following assessment he was judged to be mildly mentally retarded and at the age of four years, he was referred to a residential preschool centre for mentally handicapped children. Gradually he lost many of his behavioural disturbances and became a self-confident and happy boy. In two years, he was attending a normal kindergarten with above average achievement. When nearly seven years old, he left the school to be adopted by parents overseas. His growth performance during his time in school is shown in Figure 1, once again showing excellent "catch-up" growth.

Comment

Psycho-social influences probably constitute the single most common cause of growth failure in developed parts of the world. Its underlying pathophysiological basis has yet to be fully worked out but it likely represents the end point of several processes, most significant being lack of food from a blunted appetite and a mild depression of endocrine function.[2] These two case histories dramatically illustrate the severe stunting of stature that can occur in children who are socially and emotionally deprived early on in their lives, existing alongside other well-recognized psychological

Figure 1. Catch-up Growth in Height in the Two Children. Upper (*Case 2*), Lower (*Case 1*). 0–0 Points of Admission to and Discharge from the Residential Preschool Centre.

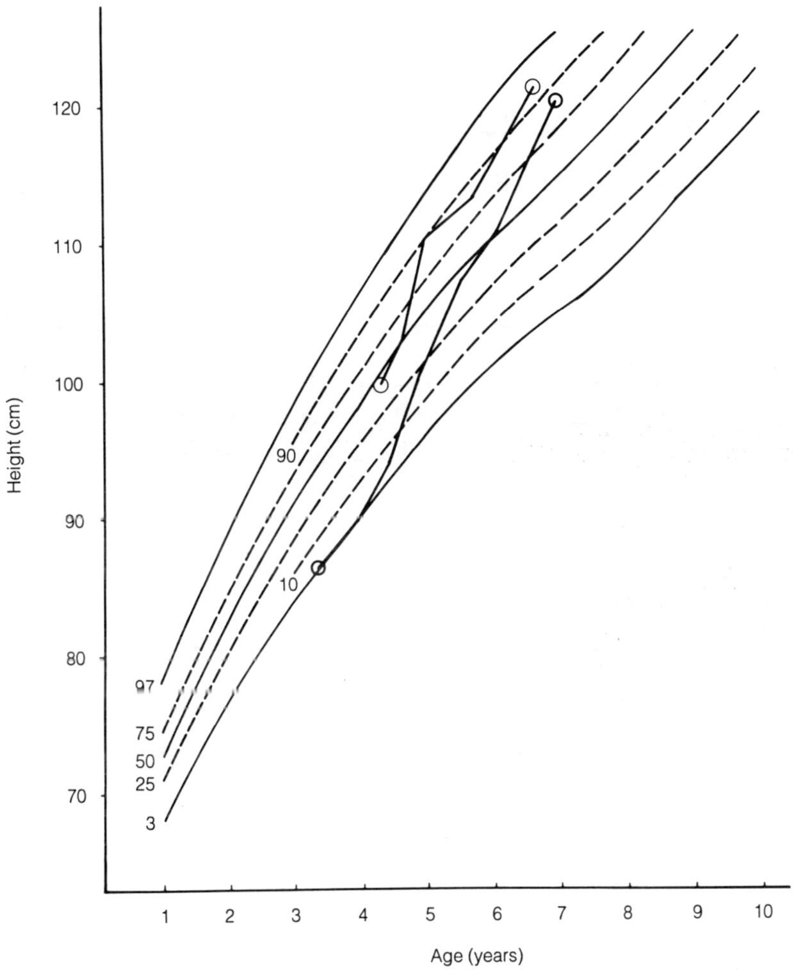

problems of apathy, submission, sleep disturbances, slow learning etc.[2] As important, but less well-documented, is the demonstration that the regular measurement of height is a very important part of the ongoing assessment of these children during their rehabilitation in order to provide an objective marker of their well-being. By somehow reversing the complex nutritional/endocrine changes attendant on deprivation, a happier psycho-social environment was able to allow recovery of the growth of the two children. Regular measurement of height and its accurate documentation on a growth chart should be mandatory for all children living in special institutions and orphanages.

Acknowledgements

I thank Miss J. Lee and Miss F. Lau for preparing the manuscript.

References

1. King, J. M., and Taitz, L. S. Catch Up Growth Following Abuse. *Arch Dis Child*, 1985; 60:1,152–54.
2. MacCarthy, D. The Effects of Emotional Disturbance and Deprivation on Somatic Growth. In Davis, J. A., and Dobbing, J., eds., *Scientific Foundations in Paediatrics* (2nd edition). London: William Heinemann Medical Books Ltd., 1981; 54–73.

Part Two

Medical Education

7

Neuro-developmental Handicap in the Paediatric Curriculum: An Experience from a New Medical School in Hong Kong

The Welsh Paediatric Journal, 1990; 2:4–8

Summary

This article describes the approach to, and the content of, the teaching about neuro-developmental problems to paediatric students in the new Faculty of Medicine of The Chinese University of Hong Kong. Especially emphasized in this programme of instruction are the origins, spectrum and presentation of these disorders; the importance of prevention; the concept of multiple-system handicap and multi-disciplinary assessment and management; the roles of doctors and other professional workers; the medical, social and educational problems of the handicapped; the importance of communication with the handicapped child. The broad aim of this teaching was to prepare the ground for the future doctor, whether in hospital or community practice, to deal sensitively and competently with the handicapped child and his/her family.

Introduction

Mental handicap and other neuro-developmental disorders of childhood are assuming increasing importance as personal, community and social problems in all parts of the world, affluent and poor alike. Yet in general, medical curricula are slow to accommodate this reality into educational goals: the emphasis in medical faculties continuing in the main to rest heavily on more immediately interesting and glamorous areas of hospital-based medicine. A recent article[1] has provided examples of a continuing neglect of mental handicap in the medical curricula of British medical schools: a median allocation of only 12 hours of curriculum time being reported in 23 medical schools surveyed, showing little change from the 11.5 hours reported ten years earlier in a similar survey.[2] Contrast this experience with the many laborious hours spent by students in operating theatres and hanging around business ward rounds awaiting the pearls of wisdom and knowledge to drop from the "masters lips"! Yet who can deny the impressive contribution to paediatric morbidity made by mental handicap, the cerebral palsies, visual and hearing problems, behavioural disturbances and learning disabilities, and the continuing indifference and insensitivity shown by so many doctors to the handicapped child and his/her family.

In Hong Kong, doctors have also had to become more aware about problems of neuro-developmental handicap as the ravages of poverty, undernutrition and communicable diseases have in one generation been largely eliminated. This chapter describes the approach to the teaching of mental handicap and other neuro-developmental problems to medical students in the course of their paediatric instruction in the Department of Paediatrics of The Chinese University of Hong Kong where I worked from 1982 to 1989. I offer this contribution since Paediatricians throughout Wales are committed to teaching medical students about neuro-developmental problems and I thought they might be interested to read an account of such a teaching programme in a part of the world where, until recently, the management of neuro-developmental disability was not a major priority in the face of many and more immediate health concerns.

Background: The Paediatric Curriculum

The Faculty of Medicine of The Chinese University of Hong Kong graduated its first batch of students in 1985. The clinical section of the faculty is based in the Prince of Wales Hospital, a 1,600-bed hospital in Sha Tin, a new urban development in the New Territories serving the comprehensive medical needs of nearly one million people. The medical curriculum, extending over five years, follows the traditional British model with teaching mostly subject based with varied amounts of horizontal and vertical collaborative instruction. Basic science preparation takes place in the first two pre-clinical years. The major bulk of paediatric teaching takes place during a ten-week module in the second clinical year where it rotates with three similar lengthened modules of Obstetrics and Gynaecology, Community and Family Medicine, and Psychiatry. Prior to these rotations is a two-week core lecture course at the beginning of the academic year which is shared with the Department of Obstetrics and Gynaecology and when lectures on common paediatric topics are given.

The broad aim of our paediatric teaching was to provide an overview of the medical problems of children with special relevance to Hong Kong and Southeast Asia — their origins, presentation, management and prevention. We took every opportunity to emphasize the holistic approach to clinical practice, striving to keep the balance between acute and chronic problems of childhood. Teaching about normal growth and development took place in the second pre-clinical year through a joint course of lectures with the Department of Anatomy. Further insight into normal childhood development was gained through an Integrated Family Follow-up project where, in the first week of pre-clinical studies, students were allocated to new-born baby and then subsequent follow-up visits were made at regular intervals to the family home for the next three years. A report on this experience has to be prepared and presented, summarizing among other things the health and psychosocial development of the young infant, physical growth and social interactions, and adjustments which take place within the family following the arrival of a new child.

Instruction in Neuro-developmental Handicap

Our broad aim was simple: to prepare the ground for the future doctor to be able to deal sensitively and competently with the neuro-developmental handicapped and their families whether as general practitioner, paediatrician, psychiatrist, casualty doctor or any other medical practitioner in hospital and community alike. (Behavioural and learning disorders were dealt with during the teaching of child psychiatry and are not dealt with further in this chapter.)

Teaching about children with neuro-developmental handicap was spread throughout the ten-week course, being sold conceptually to the students as problems caused by underlying irreversible interference with normal brain growth early in development with the many and diverse pathophysiological mechanisms and aetiological roots determining the functional outcome and pattern of developmental abnormality. Also emphasized and contrasted with many of the other paediatric "system disorders" was that the assessment and management of neuro-developmental disability nearly always demands a multi-disciplinary approach where, in various combinations, clinical psychologists, paediatricians, physiotherapists, teachers, occupational therapists, speech therapists, surgeons etc., all work together as a team to identify and manage the problems in order to lessen as far as possible the impact of an irreversible insult to the developing brain. Students were made to appreciate the wide interface that various management programmes have with the community. Most handicapped children in Hong Kong are looked after outside the mainstream of hospital wards and clinics. A large number attend special schools, many residential, where attention is given to their education, medical and social needs.

The following aspects of neuro-developmental handicap were touched upon during the paediatric course:

1. definitions, epidemiology, origins, presentation and prevention;
2. identifying and assessing (by various attainment tests) children with handicap;
3. the concept of multiple-system handicap and the principles of multi-disciplinary assessment and management;
4. the roles of the many professional workers involved with handicapped children;
5. communication with handicapped children; and
6. the particular role of the non-specialist doctor with the handicapped child.

Teaching Methods

Epidemiology, Origins and Presentation of Handicap

These aspects were covered principally in two lectures during the two-week core lecture course at the start of the second clinical year. These lectures encompassed in particular common neuro-developmental disorders, developmental assessment and the specific role of the doctor in dealing with the mentally handicapped. In later visits to a special school for mentally handicapped children, a maternal and child health (MCH) clinic, child assessment centre, cerebral palsy clinic and a hospital neonatal follow-up clinic, opportunity was further taken to demonstrate and explain the causes of handicap.

Early Identification and Initial Assessment

Many neuro-developmental disabilities are identified in the course of routine programmes of surveillance of health and development in the 47 MCH clinics throughout Hong Kong, and during the follow-up clinics. Students had one visit to an MCH clinic lasting a day and two visits to an afternoon neonatal "Follow-up" baby clinic.

The Multi-disciplinary Approach to Assessment and Management

Teaching this aspect took place in a single-day visit to a Child Assessment Centre in Kowloon. When our curriculum was initially planned in 1983, the original intention behind this visit was for students to see several children followed from their initial presentation with suspected or proven handicap through the various sequences of assessment — medical, psychological, physical, education, special sense, etc. — ending with a "case conference" in which recommendations are made regarding management in time of the identified problems. This ideal came to pose increasing logistic problems because of the considerable clinical demands made on this single Assessment Centre which served the needs of an estimated population of nearly three million. What came to be given instead to the students was (far from ideal) a general lecture in the Centre followed by a tour simply to show what an Assessment Centre is. In 1990–91, there will be a newly functioning Child Assessment Centre close to the Prince of Wales Hospital and this will hopefully improve the teaching of the multi-disciplinary approach to handicap.

In order to plug this temporary gap in our teaching, a multi-disciplinary neuro-developmental clinic was set up in the hospital once a month, coordinated by myself, in which there was physiotherapy, occupational therapy, social work and paediatric input. Children seen were those who had been referred to me and who, instead of seeing them in a general clinic, were brought to this combined clinic. The educational emphasis was not on fact, syndromes and signs but on the principles of a collaborative approach so that the role of the paediatrician and other health professionals could be better identified and understood. This combined approach was further consolidated when our students attended on two occasions a Cerebral Palsy Clinic run jointly by a physiotherapist, orthopaedic surgeon and a paediatrician.

Roles of Other Professional Workers

Students in groups of 3 to 4 attended for one day the Occupational Therapy and Physiotherapy Departments, which together make up the hospital rehabilitation unit, to gain insight into the roles of these workers in the management and rehabilitation of neuro-developmental disability. This further served as a model to emphasize the importance of paramedical health professionals in the long-term care of the handicapped child. Here the students also had "hands on" experience playing with children while they were undergoing therapy, many of whom were in a toy library, and they were able at the same time to take the opportunity to remind themselves of some of the physical signs of cerebral palsy.

Social, Educational and Medical Aspects of Handicap

Handicap generates many social, behavioural and educational consequences to the child and family. As if it is not enough for children to suffer handicap, they are also troubled by medical problems, many shared in common with normal children. The most severe and demanding of these medical problems are convulsive disorders and behavioural disturbances. In Hong Kong, many handicapped children still spend much of their time in residential schools as weekly, and in a small minority, full-time boarders; this arrangement contributes additional problems of communicable diseases (especially diarrhoea), skin infestations, respiratory infections, etc. Students were taught about these problems during a visit to a special school for mentally handicapped children.

In this allocation, students (3 to 4 at a time) spent one day in Pinehill Village in Tai Po, a large urban development situated about five miles from our hospital. The Village is operated by the Hong Kong Association for the Mentally Handicapped and is government-subvented. There are five projects in the Village which provide both residential and non-residential

Figure 1. Happy Children in Pinehill Village.

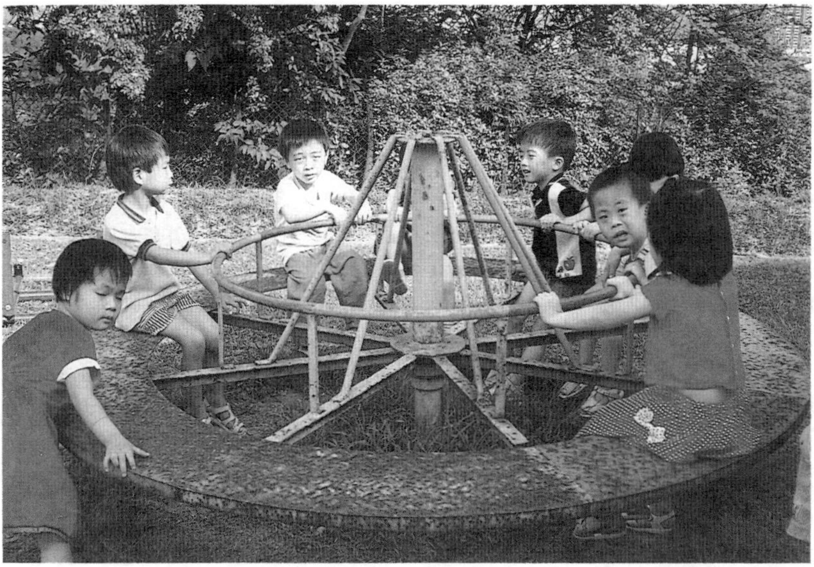

facilities for nearly 300 children with mild, moderate and severe mental handicap with age groups ranging from 3 to 16 years who are looked after there (Figure 1). If students so wished, they could spend the following Saturday morning in the Village. In the same location, there is also an Advanced Training Centre (a weekly residential Training Centre) aimed at providing vocational training for mildly or moderately mentally handicapped youths aged 16 to 20 years. Here the opportunity is provided to earn a skill (metal work, carpentry, assembly of industrial products, cotton work, knitting, etc.) to prepare the young adults for later gainful employment in the community. The visit to this Training Centre was vital for our students since it was able to show them that the handicapped are real people many of whom can and do contribute to the workforce of the community.

Students were given little formal instruction at the Village. Instead, they were encouraged to mix with the children, play with them, sit with them during their classes and meal times, and to learn a little about problems in communicating with them. They also "sat in" during a medical surgery for these children which I conducted once a week to be taught something about their medical problems and to appreciate some other responsibilities that doctors have towards the mentally handicapped. I emphasized to the students that without enjoying the best possible physical health, these children can never achieve their optimal development potential. In most Western countries, the medical care of mentally handicapped children in special schools is usually the responsibility of community doctors working closely with the hospital services. In parts of the world where paediatric community services have yet to be developed, and Hong Kong is of this category, alternative arrangements to look after this physical well-being of these institutionalized children must evolve. To have paediatricians regularly visiting these places is one such model that is being encouraged in Hong Kong.

I must stress that the principal purpose of the visit to this special school was not to make the student learn the physical signs and symptoms of handicap and details of frequently associated rare syndromes (dearly loved by generations of students and teachers alike!). It was intended simply to provide them a glimpse, however brief and superficial, into the world of problems of children with neuro-developmental handicap (Figure 2), the immense demands made on their families and all workers who have to care for them, and the medical and behavioural problems that are encountered. The students had to understand that with suitable care, children, however handicapped, can progress and live with dignity. Regretted was that so little time in the medical curriculum was made available for such visits which, providing they were carefully structured and planned with clear objectives given at the outset, I considered extremely valuable. Indeed, I would ideally have liked other visits to have been arranged so that the students saw a wider range of children with mental and physical disability. With chronic disability emerging as an increasing problem in Hong Kong, such visits are needed.

The experience of spending time with these children and obtaining some insight into their problems also helped students appreciate the need, wherever possible, to PREVENT the occurrence of handicap and how the doctor can help in this regard. At the same time, seeing many happy and loved children with Down's Syndrome also made the students think long, hard and uncomfortably about the ethics of prenatal diagnosis, the mechanical and technical aspects they would have been taught in their obstetric module.

Figure 2. A Visit of Medical Students to Pinehill Village Where Casual Interaction between the Students and the Mentally Handicapped Was Made Possible.

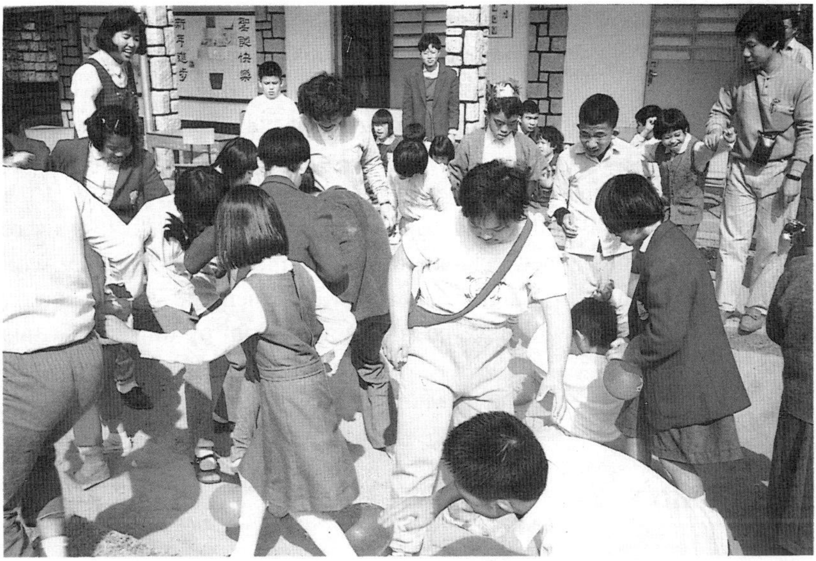

Communication with the Mentally Handicapped

Children with mental handicap share with children of normal intelligence the usual ailments of childhood. They have also to communicate their symptoms to doctors and also to be examined by them. Those severely retarded rely solely on their parents and nurses to somehow communicate their symptoms. But mild-grade children will often be expected to tell the doctor themselves, though in very rudimentary a fashion. This they always find very difficult. They become anxious and flustered when seeing a doctor and are usually overwhelmed. At the same time, doctors themselves all too often adopt a far from empathetic attitude to these children, many feeling profoundly embarrassed at their encounter.

To help these children express themselves and to improve their confidence (a very important aspect given that many of these children as later adults will be employed in sheltered workshops, advanced training centres where they will be considered part of the community), the medical students "role-played" as doctors in a special evening clinic, asking questions about their health and giving them a simple physical examination. In this way the children were given a "medical experience" so that when they were really to have later symptoms of illness, then it was to be hoped that these experiences would help them a little to communicate better and make them less nervous. In turn, medical students also benefited since the experiences provide them with an opportunity to talk to children with a mental disability.

On the whole, doctors are not very good at talking to mentally handicapped persons. They feel awkward and embarrassed, an attitude that relays itself to parents as one often of callous indifference. Indeed, if the single day in Pinehill Village did no more than make future doctors aware that mentally handicapped persons are real human beings, sharing with those more fortunate the same needs and wants, then one very important educational objective will have been achieved. I am optimistic that this contact, however short, will have its effect in later years to help lift the veil of ignorance, indifference and insecurity.

Conclusion

With such a short time available in the Medical Curriculum, all we were able to give our medical students was an overview of the problems and principles underlying the management of handicapped children and a glimpse into the harsh and unfair realities of their world and that which they share with their families. If at the end of the paediatric module students emerged more aware of the existence of these children and had begun to appreciate the immense challenges facing those who have to care for them and their families, then some of the broad principal objectives would have been achieved.

Unlike topic teaching of the "system" disorders that more readily lends itself to instruction in hospital clinics and ward rounds, teaching about neuro-developmental handicap, by the very nature of the diversity of its causes, manifestations and multi-disciplinary management has inevitably to be fragmented. Clearly defined aims must therefore be given to students at the start of their course so that they can begin to piece together this complex jigsaw puzzle. Medical students everywhere I have taught have difficulty in appreciating that many professional workers need be involved in the total care of these children. In such a complex multi-disciplinary area, the specific role of the doctor is discerned by students with difficulty: they see the non-specialist doctor's responsibilities as often peripheral to other disciplines with help, when given, being usually more educational and social than medical. Coming to terms with this peripheral role they often found difficulty. I hope that the all too brief exposure given to our students of neuro-developmental problems of children during their paediatric teaching would have begun to help them to sort out this role.

Acknowledgements

Of the many people who over the years have helped me gain some understanding of the world of the handicapped child and the importance of allowing the medical student a glimpse into this world, I would like to single out Miss Nora Wong, Superintendent of Pinehill Village, who through her selfless devotion to the cause of mentally handicapped children, shows by supreme example how the dignity of these people can always preserved.

This teaching programme would not have been possible without the enthusiastic and willing assistance from many colleagues in the Prince of Wales Hospital Rehabilitation Unit, Arran Street Child Assessment Centre, Lek Yuen MCH clinic, hospital out-patient clinics, Pinehill Village. To these colleagues I extend my sincere thanks and appreciation.

References

1. Hollins, S. How Mental Handicap Is Taught in U.K. Medical Schools. *Med Teacher*, 1988; 10:289–96.
2. Pilkington, T. Teaching Medical Students about Mental Handicap. *Dev Med Child Neurol*, 1977; 19:652–58.

8

So Little Time to Learn So Much: An Educational Challenge to Undergraduate Clinical Teaching

The Hong Kong Journal of Paediatrics, 1991; 8:61–71

It behoves well, at a time of growing interest and concern about many aspects of continuing postgraduate professional medical education, to remind ourselves of some of its preparatory foundations — notably medical education in the undergraduate years. In this chapter, I concern myself with one aspect, namely some views on clinical education in general.

My comments are a synthesis of impressions gathered over nearly twenty years of involvement in undergraduate medical education. They are intended as neither exhaustive nor all-embracing but I hope they will provoke some response and maybe even prick one or two consciences! I would also like to make clear from the outset that these thoughts are mine alone and do not necessarily represent those of any medical faculty with which I have been associated.

Changing Times, Changing Expectations

Undergraduate clinical medical teaching continues the process of preparation for a lifetime's vocational commitment to one of the many disciplines of "medicine": to produce doctors, competent professionals, who can provide health care.[1] For a long time, spanning centuries, the major emphasis in clinical education was on "training"; dogmatic instruction followed by practical supervision until competence was achieved. In Britain and France even several hundred years ago, "... students, or the apprenticeship physicians, were walked through the hospital wards by the master from bed to bed, watching him at work, assisting him at this and at that and noting the words that fell from his lips."[2] Diagnosis was usually by "pattern recognition" of illness and management policies followed rigid set rules. Early medical curricula expected a graduating doctor to be immediately proficient in medicine, surgery and midwifery without further vocational training.

How times have changed! The educational emphasis is now to provide the medical student with an education on broader and more general lines — as first enunciated many years ago in the 1944 *Goodenough Report*: "To instruct less and to educate more: to encourage individual critical thought, initiative and self learning." To produce graduates who can apply scientific biomedical principles in order to manage health problems. "To produce an educated man who would become qualified by postgraduate training" (*Todd Report*). The view now widely held is that clinical experience and specific skills will be acquired largely after graduation. Basic medical training (the undergraduate period along with the pre-registration year) is not, to state the obvious, intended to train specialists but instead to provide doctors by the time of full registration with the necessary knowledge, clinical skills and behavioural attitudes in order to provide a basis for early supervised practice or furthest vocational training.

The young doctor now enters a world very different from that of many of their teachers:

1. Patients' expectations are much greater. They (quite rightly) demand more explanation of their problems and better care.
2. The mystique of the laying on of hands is fortunately disappearing (though many doctors dislike a challenge to their mystical supremacy).
3. The management of clinical problems by more than one professional is now far more the rule than the exception.
4. Diagnostic and therapeutic tools are not only more powerful, but in many ways and especially in regard to diagnostic tools are becoming increasingly more non-invasive, more open to abuse in their request.
5. There is worldwide clamour by the public to achieve a better balance between technological advance and humane care, so concerned are many with erratic harnessing of medical technological advances.

6. Ethical, moral and legal consequences of, and associations with, clinical problems intrude far more into decision-making, paralleling the increasing complexity of our society. With financial resources available for medical care being scrutinized for cost-effectiveness, there is now a need as never before to more efficiently rationalize the deployment of available resources, both manpower and technical. With an almost bottomless pit of armamentaria to deal with medical problems, an allocation of priorities in medical care, usually an unpalatable matter for debate, has to be made. Such choices will often have to be between provision of "exciting" medical care on the one hand (kidney transplantation, *in vitro* fertilization, ventilatory support for premature babies, etc.) with care of an increasing number of chronic disabled on the other (geriatric care, neuro-developmental handicap, etc.). A better balance between hospital and community care will somehow have to be found.
7. The gap between what can be achieved through medical technology and what is actually achieved is widening, not narrowing.
8. With modern travel the world is now "much smaller." Awareness of medical problems in parts of the world far removed from an individual's personal base is now no longer of academic interest alone. The bite of mosquito during a safari holiday in Africa can several weeks later end up as malaria in Hong Kong.
9. Computers are permeating all aspects of medical care — record-keeping, data analysis, audit, diagnostic and therapeutic assistance. Effects of these introductions on personal confidentiality and the practice of medicine are considerable and not always for the best. Sometimes the patient comes second, being lost in welter of kilobytes!
10. Famines, high endemicity of chronic malnutrition often interspersed with epidemics of infectious diseases, deplorable socio-economic conditions that have their roots in gross inequalities between rich and poor countries are, through regular portrayals of visual media, increasingly part of the consciences of the fortunate.
11. Respite care and rehabilitation, and not necessarily cure, are inevitably being more and more demanded in the developed regions of the world as the population pyramid shifts and an increasing

number of children survive with multiple neuro-developmental disability.

12. The undergraduate student has now to become much more aware of some of the wider issues of medicine which will help to evaluate and go some way to satisfy the health requirements of the community they will later serve. Three major issues can be highlighted. First, an awareness of the many changes which have taken place in the pattern of illness in which problems of malnutrition and infectious diseases have, to a large extent, been replaced by problems whose origins lie in behavioural patterns, the environment, personal lifestyle (e.g. diet, drugs, alcohol, socio-economic factors) and often unrealistic expectations of longevity. Second, an appreciation of complex interactions which exist between socio-economic factors and illness: how illness can be caused, or aggravated, by social influences and how illness can itself affect patterns of social behaviour in the patient, family and community. Included in this will also be an introduction to the interface the practice of medicine has with moral, legal and ethical issues. Third, an insight into the medical needs of *populations* as well as of individuals, in both the developing as well as the developed world.

These are only some reasons why today's undergraduate clinical syllabus has become so complex and overburdened. As never before there appears to the student a bottomless pit of knowledge to acquire. Medical curricula have somehow to adapt to these changes and select for instruction that body of subject matter necessary to understand health problems in their widest sense. Regrettably, though, a prominent feature of all too many medical schools is a resistance to change. Yet those of us who are concerned with undergraduate medical education must ensure that graduates have been suitably prepared to face these new and varied challenges with the insight to themselves recognize, accept and implement changes which might at any time be considered necessary. However, this cannot all be achieved before graduation. The seeds can only be sown in the undergraduate years — their germination and later flourishing must await continuing professional education in the postgraduate years. Indeed, I view the undergraduate years as an aperitif to the major meal of a lifetime's updating of biomedical knowledge and clinical skills. As a developmental analogy, the short but vital prenatal period anticipates a long postnatal period of development! Pursuing the analogy further, damaging influences early on can permanently affect later development.

Teaching: A Third Fiddle?

At a time when the educational challenge has never been more exciting (or difficult), it is disappointing that teaching has come to play very much a third fiddle of emphasis to clinical care and research in many medical schools. Learning continues to take place all too often as a haphazard osmosis. How many medical teachers read journals of medical education to improve their teaching skills? An audit of this activity would be interesting! If our standard of clinical care and research were to be the equivalent to our teaching, I fear patient morbidity would be high and few articles would be published in scientific journals. I remember too well the many hours I spent as a student on ward rounds eagerly awaiting the pearl to drop from the lips of the Master! When it came, if ever it came, either I was too tired or too far away to hear it. When it did arrive, it was often totally inappropriate to my level of learning, serving more to impress than to educate. Similarly, the many hours on my feet in operating theatres seeing parts of people, machines, blood and viscera and all to what avail? Have times changed much? I leave it to the reader to decide.

Excellence and enthusiasm in teaching need to contribute more than they do to career advancement. But this is difficult when there is no measurable recognition of its importance. Medical faculties the world over are currently very preoccupied with research accountability and productivity, both of which of course have essential academic functions. But at the same time faculties have also to apply themselves to help redress some of the imbalances between teaching and research activities.

Educational Goals

Out of complex web of educational needs, we have somehow to unravel some important goals in the teaching of clinical medicine. Stated simply, I believe these have as their main aim the ability of the student to identify, analyse and manage clinical problems in order to provide the fundamentals of effective, efficient and humane patient care.

The Acquisition of Knowledge

During the clinical years, students should gain a balanced appreciation of the origins, pathology, clinical presentation, principles of management and outcome of the physical and mental problems which afflict the human from conception through fetal life and birth into infancy, childhood, adolescence, adulthood, the child-bearing years and old age.

In its totality medicine has to be recognized as a science, humanely practised and deeply rooted in the basic biological and social sciences (Figure 1). The approach of its teachers should be broad and holistic — looking at health from both individual and community perspectives. The importance of the pre-clinical years of basic sciences (in the "conventional" medical curriculum) in providing an understanding of the structure and function of the human body, along with an appreciation of man's activities and roles in society, cannot be stressed too much. Yet without this corpus of knowledge, illness and its management will be poorly understood and the

Figure 1. A Preterm Baby Being Ventilated. In Its Totality, Medicine Has to Be Recognized as a Science Humanely Practised and Deeply Rooted in the Basic Biological and Social Sciences.

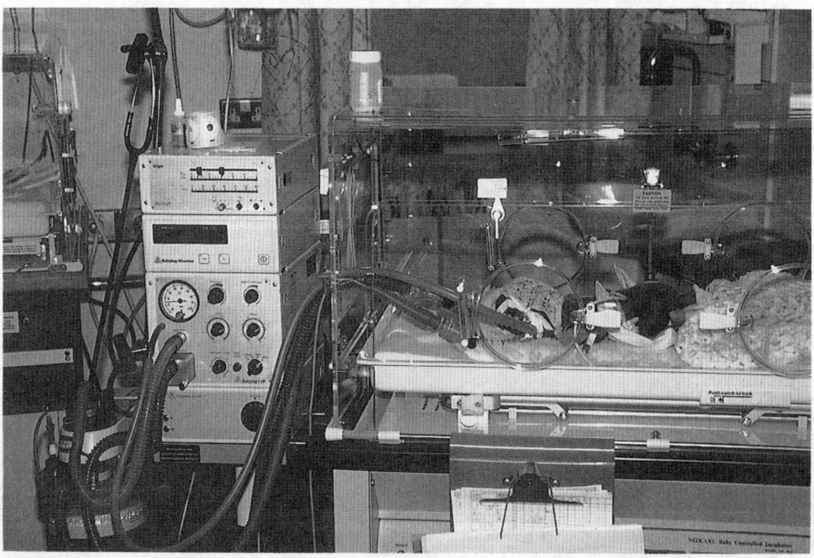

clinical years have little meaning and cannot be used to their fullest potential. Attempts by clinical teachers to erode the vitality and indispensability of the basic sciences have to be counteracted. So that students can be introduced to the mental discipline of using their knowledge of the basic sciences to work out the clinical features of disordered structure and function, every opportunity should be taken for interdisciplinary teaching between the clinical and pre-clinical departments. This continues to be an educational challenge that remains poorly explored in many faculties. Many clinical teachers fail to appreciate the value and importance of the basic sciences and this attitude of denigration is often passed onto the student. At the same time, many in the basic sciences fail to recognize that the need of medical students do differ from those in pure science streams. These bilateral misconceptions often lead to disturbed and irrelevant teaching and a sense of frustration by students and clinical teachers.

Clinical Skills

Problem-based Learning

The essential skill to be acquired in the clinical years, ideally through a guided apprenticeship on the wards and not wayward opportunism, is the clinical method: the identification (through accurate data collection), analysis and management of clinical problems efficiently, effectively and humanely. On the whole, medical students have little difficulty in acquiring a sound basis of biomedical knowledge, but their facility to acquire, synthesize and record clinical information obtained through the history and examination using this knowledge, the clinical reasoning process, is often disproportionately weak. This is borne out in my experience by the frequent occurrence of a "shift to the left" of the curve for performance in clinical examinations compared with performance in written tests of knowledge and factual recall. In many instances, blame for this weakness cannot be attributed to the students themselves. Does it indicate an inappropriate harshness, unreal expectations and too little thought in our method of clinical assessment? Might it simply uncover poor teaching of bedside clinical skills? Does it mean we are paying too much attention in our teaching to the acquisition of biomedical facts and not to their clinical application and relevance?

There needs to emerge a better understanding of what the clinical model is all about. Patient problems at the bedside, clinic and surgery should be used more to teach the principles of problem identification and solving than, as is too often done, to simply give "facts" which can equally well, if not better, be found in up-to-date textbooks and journals. More time should be spent promoting clinical reasoning skills than subject-orientated authoritative teaching. Teachers should find suitable clinical models to give students the opportunity to use their critical thinking skills to develop clinical judgement and independent learning. The well-worked up clinical case history around an actual patient is an unsurpassed model but one too often abused and inappropriately used.[3] Arguably it provides the best example of problem-based learning. It is worthwhile recalling what was written 300 years ago in the Leyden (Holland) School:

> The method adopted was for students first of all to examine the patient on his complaint, then for each one to state his view upon the nature, causes, symptoms, prognosis, and treatment of the disease and, last of all, for the professor to confirm the correct opinion, to confute erroneous ones, and to add explanation when required.[2]

Ideas put forward by Elstein and others on generating competing diagnostic hypotheses from the earliest presentation of a clinical problem and subsequently tested by the clinical method as the major determinant of effective problem-solving need to be given more exposure.[4] Problem identification and analysis using this method should be encouraged in preference to the more ritualistic gathering of data, as is the traditional approach.

During ward rounds and clinical seminars emphasis should be given to basics and much less time (and this is an all too common failing) discussing issues which, though interesting for the teacher (and indeed often for the student), are not really relevant to undergraduate need. The problem-based approach, as initially proposed by Weed,[5] where diagnoses are dissected into their component parts and managed could be used more as a structure to improve clinical reasoning skills. Greater order would thereby be introduced into the science of the clinical method, which is all too often chaotic, with recognition of problems and their diagnosis more by blind guesswork and intuition than by reasoned argument. As a consequence, our practice of medicine is often slovenly and shoddy, a salutary observation bearing in mind the immense costs involved in training. There is no better example of this than that of laboratory and imaging aids used towards diagnosis.

The Abuse of Investigations

The principles underlying a responsible, critical and intelligent approach to the use of investigative options of clinical management need to be regularly inculcated. Unfortunately, as doctors we are not good at this. Excessive and inappropriate investigation (costly, often uncomfortable and not always without hazard to the patient) are common the world over and in all disciplines and regrettably point to misunderstanding of the whole essence of the clinical method. Nothing draws attention more to the remarkable homogeneity of our profession than the wanton abuse of laboratory and other diagnostic aids! This point was vividly brought home to me by an American paediatric colleague bemoaning the fact that in their part of the world, patients were seen only after tests had been done!

I would like to see the term "routine" investigations removed from our clinical vocabulary. I never cease to be surprised by the excessive number of investigations requested as part of a "diagnostic" work-up. Bad as we paediatricians might be in this regard, colleagues in adult medicine are even worse. May it simply reflect the size of adult veins that craves penetrance! To begin to overcome this waste of valuable resources, it has to be better understood that the history and examination are as much a part of the investigative progress as are those laboratory and image-based. Conceptually there is no difference between the stethoscope and chest X-ray: both are investigative tools. Perhaps the only way to improve matters is the publication of a monthly audit, by departments, of investigations requested and circulated to other departments for their comment. Even to offer incentives to departments to save money — which they themselves can spend — through the discriminating use of further diagnostic methods. A difficult educational challenge but one that has to be met.

Communication

The final component of the clinical method, and the one which in many ways is the most difficult to be learned by the student and most poorly taught by most medical teachers, is the ability to listen and talk to patients and their families about their problems and to be able to communicate intelligently and coherently with other professional workers (medical and other). This aspect is too often neglected in the undergraduate curriculum — it is assumed that students will just happen to learn about it. Some students are naturally good communicators, but most learn by first recognizing that communication is an essential part of the clinical method, no less important than the clinical reasoning process. It is up to them to improve their communication skills by guided instruction, the use of video recordings, peer emulation, etc. The General Medical Council in Britain is at the present time laying particular emphasis on the better teaching of communication skills. Faculties need to respond to this by paying more attention to this in medical curriculum.

Poor communication leaves a patient in fear and uncertainty. Perhaps if greater effort was put into this aspect of learning by their teachers, doctors would be better skilled in this aspect. Every newly graduated batch of doctors may seem on the surface more sophisticated in relation to knowledge, to new methods of diagnosis and treatment and knowledgeable about details of rare and esoteric disorders to such an extent that their older colleagues might on occasions feel scientifically inadequate and inferior! Yet it is the use to which this knowledge is put, and the attitude in dealing with patients, that is the key to the good practice of clinical medicine. More interest is often shown in the disease itself than in the person suffering that disease. Yet recent research has shown that the ways doctors interact with their patients have a major effect on the clinical interview, compliance and satisfaction with treatment. A more conscious effort must be made to encourage students to sit down more and talk to patients and in so doing come to real terms with the problem instead of locking themselves in the library learning an endless list of diagnosis of little benefit to anyone. Knowledge which cannot be used is after all useless.

Assessment and Examination

In most medical schools, too little attention is given to assessment and evaluation of educational attainments. It seems to be assumed that not only is a good doctor a competent teacher but also an able assessor of skills and knowledge. This is far from being the case. Some may say that since most doctors are reasonably competent in their work, the means (the educational system they have passed through) has been justified by the end (effective and efficient patient care). Yet can we be that complacent? How effective and efficient really is this care? Patients regularly complain of rude and unsympathetic doctors. As I mentioned, a huge amount of money is wasted in profligate over investigation (which is never seriously audited) and recommendations for inappropriately costly treatments. Much of our practice of medicine is shoddy and second rate. Indeed, were it not for the human body's remarkable capacity to so often right itself in the face of inappropriate medical onslaught, the outcome of therapeutic management would be less successful! So the way in which we assess our students should not engender complacency.

It is now well established that a student's pattern of learning and hence later medical practice is heavily influenced by the content and method of their examinations. So do our methods of assessment truly measure these important professional qualities that are so often lacking in the medical profession? I sometimes have my doubts. Is it not time for Medical Schools in general to accept greater responsibility to instruct its clinical teachers in methods of teaching and assessment? So complex now are medical curricula that a Department of Medical Education, fully staffed and equipped, should *ideally* be part of each Medical Faculty.

If as it is generally agreed that the broad aims of undergraduate medical clinical teaching are to teach the fundamentals of understanding, identifying, assessing clinical problems and their management in an effective, humane and efficient way, then assessment should require demonstration by students of such principles. Conventional assessment is undertaken by various combinations of written tests (multiple-choice questions, data and slide analysis questions, patient management problems, essays, short notes, etc.), that are designed to test recall of fact, concepts and principles, and clinical examinations (long and short cases) to test clinical competence. But are we still falling into the trap of testing depth of knowledge (much of it irrelevant) rather than how knowledge can be used? Are we as examiners impressed more by a list of biochemical tests than with discriminatory skills students should begin to acquire as to which tests are of most value in a given clinical situation? A good doctor is one who can, in addition to effectively and efficiently manage clinical problems, give patients satisfaction by sensitively explaining the nature of the problem and its management and outcome, and be able to deal empathetically yet confidently with questions and concern that might arise. This aspect of counselling, reassurance though effective communication, is rarely touched upon in examinations. Maybe it is too difficult! Maybe examiners do not on the whole believe it worthy of assessment! Yet, should a student who proves himself knowledgeable in the language of medicine yet openly through insensitivity to a patients feelings cause embarrassment and distress be allowed to pass?

Maybe the time has arrived to re-examine our assessment methods and to ponder carefully whether our written tests and clinical examinations truly measure the competence we are seeking in our students. It is, for example, known that performance in multiple-choice questions correlates poorly with ratings of ability by clinical teachers. I am regularly impressed by young doctors whose academic records were very mediocre. Standard clinical examination performance relates poorly to observed interviewing and observational skills. Perhaps more thought should be given to the use of the Objective Structured Clinical Examination (OSCE), a more efficient tool to objectively assess essential clinical skills.

Curriculum Planning

With expansion and ever-increasing specialization within medical schools, everyone wants to have a bite of the cherry. There is often too little discussion given to whether a topic/subject lends itself more to the undergraduate or postgraduate phase of learning. Too much fact (much unnecessary) is being hurled in the direction of the student. This is wrong and leads to the cynical conclusion that the curriculum is principally for the benefit of teachers, their egos and individual departments! Indeed, fighting for curriculum time becomes for some an important clinical pastime. Imbalances in the curriculum emerge with the principal casualties being those who are most intended to benefit — the students (embryo doctors) and the community they will later serve. There is a need for greater collaboration between departments to help students integrate their knowledge — this principle should also be more widely used in the assessment process. Likewise individual departments should also accept a degree of subservience on their part to the goals of the whole course. The organization and allocation of time in the busy three clinical years of undergraduate study must take into account and reflect in a balanced way the general principles I have outlined in this chapter, encouraging at every opportunity the philosophy of collaboration, vertically in depth and horizontally in breadth, in the understanding and management of clinical problems viewed against the background of community needs.

The Faculty of Medicine of The Chinese University of Hong Kong is still making an attempt to put this ideal into practice by having a considerable amount of interdisciplinary teaching between the Departments of Community Medicine and Family Practice, Obstetrics and Gynaecology, Paediatrics and Psychiatry, all taught in 10-week modules in the second clinical year. Students at the end of the year are also examined at a Part 1 Final MB BCh in an integrated manner with written questions extending across specialty interfaces and with clinical long cases (randomly chosen from one of the four disciplines) being examined by a team of four examiners one from each discipline. What we were attempting to teach and assess was a more holistic approach to clinical medicine. I believe the experiment worked to the benefit of both students and clinical teachers.

Yet unfortunately the multiplication of departments and disciplines in medical faculties have so compartmentalized medicine as to make change often difficult to achieve. There is a need for greater integration between departments, not only clinical but also those of the basic sciences. Knowledge of basic sciences has all too often been lost, or is at least hazy, by the time the student comes to apply it to the understanding and management of illness seen in daily clinical experiences. In contrast in some of the more forward-thinking medical schools such as McMaster (Canada) and Newcastle (Australia) where teaching focuses from the outset of the undergraduate course around clinical problems, and in so doing introduce early on in the medical course the relevance and importance of scientific principles to health problems in real life, more traditional medical schools have a long way to go to more efficiently integrate the basic and applied medical sciences. Frequently, students have difficulty in remembering basic information they were given only a few months previously. This is often because teachers fail to impress on students knowledge that is or is not important and too little opportunity is taken to help students recall what they have been taught by well-planned collaborative teaching.

In our enthusiasm to prepare students for their future careers, one note of caution must be sounded: "The medical student faces the unbearable task of seeking to master an overwhelming range of knowledge and skills many of which he will never need to utilize in his career — a fact of which he is well aware as a student."[6] There is so much to learn that students will "miss the wood for the trees." It has been estimated (How? I do not know!) that medical students are expected to learn about 48,000 facts and 30,000 basic medical science concepts and an additional 53,000 clinical facts and concepts.[7] The problem becomes insoluble — how to fit an exponentially growing amount of knowledge into a fixed amount of curricular time. At the same time, there is inadequate encouragement of critical thinking. Principles have to be emphasized in preference to giving a multitude of facts. Skeletons should be provided. The flesh of knowledge can be hung on this skeleton by students themselves. Medical schools do after all take from schools academically very gifted students. The emphasis must be on acquiring those knowledge and skills that can immediately recognized by the medical student to help him/her understand and best manage medical problems effectively.

At the same time, it is also important not to overload students' time for other personal reasons. There is a tendency to overrate the capabilities of young students to cope personally with clinical problems. Many find contact with ill patients distressing (for many will probably be their first contact with serious illness and death). Indeed, depression and peculiar health fantasies are not uncommon in medical students, though few care to admit it.

Time to relax and ponder a little is as important as time directed for teaching. Some teachers, highly motivated but misguided, wish to cram into a few undergraduate years a lifetime of medical experience. They tend to lose sight of their principal objectives. I repeat again that it must also be constantly borne in mind by planners of medical curricula that the teaching programme is for students' benefit, not that of the Faculty of Medicine! Not every subject needs to be given prominence at undergraduate level. Indeed, it is the failure to grasp this principle that accounts for much of the distortions, overcrowding and imbalances which exist in so many medical courses. If it is accepted that medical education is a continuum (analogous to human life with the undergraduate period equivalent to prenatal life and postgraduate corresponding with postnatal life [birth and the final M.B. being comparable hurdles to overcome!]), some subjects lend themselves far better to postgraduate than to undergraduate study. There is also all too often an overemphasis at undergraduate level on teaching details of management. How can the student, who has never had the responsibility for actually managing a patient, and who will everyday hear senior members of medical staff argue among themselves, learn details of treatment? Details of management are more for the postgraduate. The understanding of common illnesses — reaching a differential diagnosis, understanding the principles of management and the awareness of the psychosocial consequences of illness to the patient, family and friends is for the undergraduate. Competency to practice is not now a legitimate aim in professional undergraduate medical education. The better-equipped the student with principles, the easier will it be to begin the next stage, notably to put all these educational ideals into the practice of medicine.

Conclusion

A major criticism of our profession is often not that we are insufficiently clever but that we often think ourselves too clever to spend time in listening to and talking with patients and their relatives! The practice of medicine is primarily a humanity; attitudes of thoughtfulness, humility, kindliness and humour must be fostered as early as possible. It is salutary to be again reminded about a growing fear on the part of the lay public of the power of medicine, the risk of iatrogenesis and depersonalization. Technology and computers are sometimes seen to take over from the kindly bedside manner. There is all too often dissatisfaction with the doctor and patient relationship. Patients want doctors to listen more, understand their beliefs and attitudes better, and to discuss with them their problems in language they understand. Indeed, it is this general disillusionment that has forced some academic authorities to wonder whether the very high academic standards required for entry of medical students into university might be selecting those academically more able (whatever this might mean) at the expense of those better able to declare empathy. However, compassion itself requires an innate intelligence to be able to put oneself into another person's lesser fortunate position in order to give the required empathy. To necessarily imply that care, compassion and intelligence are incompatible as sleeping partners is not only dangerous — leading perhaps to a fall in standards — but also unfounded. But it is the responsibility of teachers to ensure that these human aspects of clinical practice are introduced early on into our students thinking, and are given an equal importance to other aspects of learning in the medical curriculum.

Acknowledgements

I thank my many colleagues and medical students who over the years have allowed themselves to be used as sounding boards for many of the ideas expressed in this chapter. I thank Ruth Webber for typing this manuscript.

References

1. Cox, K. Knowledge Which Cannot Be Used Is Useless. *Med Teacher*, 1987; 9:145–59.
2. Puschmann, T. *History of Medical Education.* New York: Hafner, 1966. Quoted in Pallic, W., and Carr, D. H. The McMaster Medical Education Philosophy in Therapy, Practice and Historical Perspective. *Med Teacher*, 1987; 9:59–71.
3. Edwards, J. C., Braunan, J. R., Burgess, L., *et al.* Case Presentation Format and Clinical Reasoning: A Strategy for Teaching Medical Students. *Med Teacher*, 1987; 9:285–92.
4. Elstein, A. S., Kagon, N., Shulman, L., *et al.* Methods and Theory in the Study of Medical Inquiry. *J Med Educ*, 1972; 47:85–92.
5. Weed, L. L. *Medical Records, Medical Education and Patient Care*. Chicago: Year Book Medical Publishers, 1971.
6. Anderson, J., and Graham, A. A Problem in Medical Education: Is There an Information Overload? *Med Education*, 1980; 14:4–7.
7. Blunt, M. J., and Blizard, P. Recall and Retrieval of Anatomical Knowledge. *Br J Med Educ*, 1975; 9:225–63.

Part Three

Miscellaneous

9

*The Realities of Neonatal Practice**

Hong Kong Paediatric Society Year Book, 1983; 27–29

The spectrum of problems in the neonatal period varies throughout the world along with attitudes to, and arrangements available for, their management. Notwithstanding there do exist certain fundamental principles which underlie the practice of neonatal care wherever undertaken. It is with these that this article is concerned.

Setting the Scene

For many, neonatal paediatrics is synonymous with the care of new-born babies at risk of, or suffering from, the consequences of premature birth; afflicted by major errors of morphogenesis (congenital malformations); embarrassed by maternal illness; insulted by difficult birth or stunted by intra-uterine growth retardation. These problems together account for about 95% of deaths in the perinatal period and generate much of the neonatal workload and contribute significantly to later problems of physical and neuro-developmental disability. The demands made by sick new-born babies have provided much of the impetus for the development of neonatal intensive care methods and in so doing placed the stamp of credibility on the young subject of neonatology. It would nonetheless be a mistake to hold the view that care of the ill or potentially ill baby is all that constitutes neonatal practice. Preterm births, severe intra-partum asphyxia, major

---

* Based on a lecture given to the Hong Kong Paediatric Society in October 1982.

congenital malformations and significant growth retardation account for about 10–15% of all births. Yet, it is common practice in the first few days of life for up to 15–25% (even higher in some parts of the world depending on local arrangements for the care of the new-born) of babies to be admitted to a neonatal unit, needing a level of care greater than can be given on the usual postnatal ward. Furthermore, of normal babies on lying-in wards whose postnatal course is without major interruption, many will have minor problems such as feeding difficulties, jaundice, skin rashes, heart murmurs etc. which will need attention.

These events therefore point to the neonatal period being one of somewhat surprising morbidity. Yet, this should perhaps not be unexpected since the new-born period is after all one of unpredictable transition. Premature delivery and prenatal growth retardation remain a constant fraction of all births in spite of improved care during pregnancy. The birth process itself, even with the best perinatal care, is unpredictable with many hostile forces, both natural (the birth canal) and unnatural (methods of assisted delivery) ready to interfere with the baby's smooth entry into the world and its adjustment to postnatal life. Examination of the new-born baby will inevitably reveal its fair share of abnormalities. In the early days after birth, the baby has completely to change the method by which it derives its food, from being intravenously fed across the placenta to an enteral form of nutrition. Is it therefore surprising the number of upsets that can take place?

The scope of neonatal practice is therefore much wider than is often believed. In its totality, neonatal care should be considered a general discipline, its claim for specialty status being founded in such small persons. In itself neonatal care is no more a "specialty" than are the problems of later infancy, adolescence and adulthood although, and in common with the other epochs of childhood and adulthood, there is ample scope for specialization *within* the subject (cardiorespiratory intensive care; nutrition; neurology; neuro-developmental follow-up; surgical management of congenital abnormalities, to name but a few).

The Compartments of Neonatal Practice

Neonatal practice can for conceptual purposes be conveniently considered in five, albeit arbitrary, interrelating compartments.

Involvement with Life before Birth

Many of the problems which present in the new-born period have their origins in prenatal life (see below). It is therefore sensible and logical for paediatricians to be involved in this period. Two examples of such involvement might be:

1. Interest in the course of pregnancy and the method of delivery in certain high-risk cases (e.g. growth retardation, maternal diabetes, rhesus disease [in European populations] and hypertension).
2. A contribution to the often controversial issues of screening in the antenatal period for abnormalities of fetal development (e.g. neural tube defects, haemoglobinopathies, Down's Syndrome).

These are only two examples which serve to illustrate how paediatricians can be involved during the prenatal period. It is this involvement (paralleling that shown by obstetricians in the neonatal period) which has helped the concept of perinatal medicine to evolve — concern for the whole continuum of life before, during and in the early period after birth. In day-to-day practice, this is best achieved by paediatricians participating in, and making themselves available to, obstetric discussions on ward rounds and clinics. In terms of training, it is desirable for paediatricians to have residency experience in obstetric practice.

Birth, the New-born Examination and Normal Events of the First Week

This compartment contains the very general aspects of neonatal care which concern all babies who are born but who will not necessarily require any special attention. The great majority of new-born babies belong to this category. It is essential to provide the safest possible environment for birth: the new-born must be carefully examined to detect physical abnormalities (such as congenital dislocation of the hip) and, through metabolic screening, conditions such as phenylketonuria, hypothyroidism and glucose–6–phosphate dehydrogenase (G–6–PD) deficiency. Feeding (both breast-feeding and bottle-feeding) will often need attention as also will problems such as jaundice, skin rashes, vomiting. However mundane and trivial might appear many of these aspects of neonatal care, they are very important. If managed poorly, considerable anxiety and unnecessary suffering can be caused.

The "Problem" Baby

This compartment of neonatal care is concerned with those babies who require to be admitted to a neonatal unit. These "problem" babies fall into two categories according to whether:

1. problems are anticipated (e.g. preterm birth, baby of a diabetic mother, intra-uterine growth retardation); or
2. where problems have already declared themselves (e.g. overt congenital abnormalities, respiratory distress soon after birth, severe jaundice, convulsions).

Depending upon the criteria for admission to a neonatal unit and which will themselves often depend as much on logistic arrangements within any particular hospital as on medical need, these problem babies will amount to between 10–20% of all new-born babies. Where no facilities exist on postnatal wards for looking after even the most mundane of problems (e.g. a vomiting baby), this percentage can be as high as 30%.

The most exciting events of neonatal care usually take place in the intensive care area where the cardiorespiratory support of infants with breathing problems dominate. Equal attention must also be given to the low dependency area where babies are in the process of being weaned for discharge home. Interesting problems in this area such as growth and nutrition, infant-family interactions, criteria for discharge home, anaemia of prematurity, and jaundice, all deserve their fair share of attention. Also not to be forgotten is the care of the terminally ill baby (as for example the baby with spina bifida who is not being operated upon). Often among the most distressing of problems, these frequently present even greater challenges than are found in the more technical aspects of neonatal care.

Follow-up

The relationship between neonatal problems and their long-term outcome is the fourth compartment of neonatal care. Without such awareness, the practice of neonatal paediatrics becomes insular and inward-looking. It is my conviction that in the first place follow-up should, wherever possible, be the responsibility of the neonatal team of nurses and doctors who look after the sick neonate, working in close collaboration with specialists in the field of assessment and management of disabled children. In this way all important feedback will be obtained, necessary not only to detect early neuro-developmental handicap but also as a means to audit neonatal practices. Involvement in the follow-up clinic is especially valuable for neonatal nurses who usually have much less opportunity than doctors to learn about the consequences of the care that they provide in the early weeks after birth.

Babies followed up should include especially those, through perinatal events, at risk of neuro-developmental handicap and physical disability. Others who might need follow-up are those with minor problems found during the course of the neonatal examination (e.g. congenital dislocation of hip, heart murmurs) and during the first week (e.g. jaundice). Depending on local arrangements and attitudes, babies with major congenital anomalies (Down's Syndrome, neural tube anomalies, cleft palate) might also be seen in a follow-up clinic for the first year or so of life before continuing hospital care in the older paediatric clinic. Genetic counselling will occasionally be needed. With varying emphasis depending on the nature of the problem, follow-up care should embrace the assessment of health, growth and neuro-developmental states. Every opportunity should also be taken to encourage optimum health by advising about immunization and good feeding practices.

Support for Bereaved Parents

An important, though much neglected, compartment of neonatal practice concerns the support given to bereaved parents. There is now emerging an impression that carefully guided support in the early months after bereavement can facilitate psychological recovery after perinatal death. Helping parents who have lost their babies must be viewed as an essential part of any perinatal service. Along with psychological support, it is also important to explain, as clearly as possible, the cause of death (including results of any necropsy), along with implications for future pregnancies and any other matters which might arise. Owing to a lack of training in the subject, most paediatricians will have little knowledge of the psychopathology of bereavement and its counselling. We can still however provide a valuable service.

What is needed above all else is an open, sensitive, common sense approach which can be provided without special training, however desirable this might be. The principal questions volunteered by mothers and fathers are remarkably stereotyped: Why had the baby died? Could death have been prevented? Was it their fault? Who was to blame? Was it something they had done? What went wrong? Will it happen again? What of the future? These questions can usually be answered although sometimes difficulties will arise especially when the cause of death has its immediate origins in the intra-partum period. Ideally, the presence of an obstetrician in such a clinic is desirable. The principal function of counselling is to help dispel the many fantasies which so many parents entertain surrounding neonatal death. Indeed, much psychopathology exists in families through lack of basic explanation after neonatal (and intra-uterine) death. Parents are better able to come to terms with the death of a baby if they understand what has happened.

Most neonatal units will not have the backup social work, psychological and psychiatric services which are ideally needed to provide bereavement counselling although immediate referral of major problems to these specialists should always be possible. In some hospitals, the social work department provides invaluable support. Nonetheless, it is feasible for paediatricians to provide a service for parents which is better than exists in many hospitals. This will come about, however, only when paediatricians themselves realize its necessity. (Indeed, it is regrettable that the psychological aspects of death are so little touched on in undergraduate curricula and postgraduate training programmes.)

There is more to neonatal care than simply the technological aspects of management. The grumble that there is too little time available will inevitably be heard. Whilst in certain parts of the world this argument will certainly apply, this impediment can in many instances be overcome if the general philosophy of neonatal follow-up clinic is re-examined. Of all hospital paediatric services, the average baby follow-up clinic is probably that which has least thought devoted to it. Far too many babies are unnecessarily and uncritically followed up particularly since in so many countries there are now community surveillance programmes for health and development. Not only does this constitute considerable waste of time but for families it can be psychologically disturbing. By having carefully considered criteria for follow-up and due care given to its organization, time will become available for other matters, in this context bereavement counselling.

Conclusion

Much of my personal fascination for neonatal paediatrics lies in many interfaces shared with other branches of medicine and non-medical disciplines. The neonatal period is a true bridge linking the cloistered world of intra-uterine life with the potentially hostile existence of the "exterogestate" fetus (Figure 1). It is during this time that more than 50% of all

Figure 1. Neonates, Especially Those Born Very Prematurely, Need to Be Given Great Care Because They Have to Face Many Potential Hostilities of the "Outer" World Without the Intra-uterine Protection Previously Enjoyed in Prenatal Life.

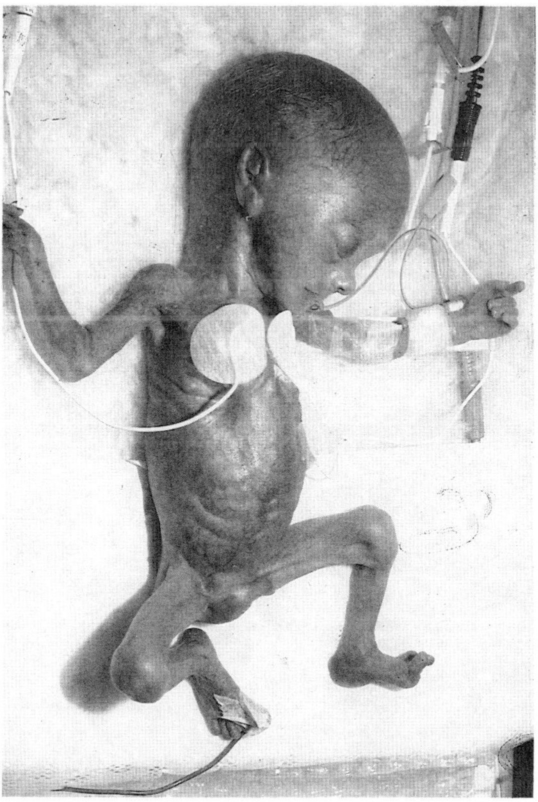

deaths in childhood take place and when the consequences of survival can be disastrous. Fortunately, increasing technological advances now make it possible for even the smallest of babies to survive, but, as a consequence, moral and ethical dilemmas are being constantly posed. With such difficult techniques having to be undertaken, the risks of iatrogenic disasters are especially real. There is therefore a need as at no other time for specializations within the subject — particularly, as I have mentioned earlier, those concerned with intensive care management. Nonetheless, I do believe that it is also important not to lose sight of the wider aspects of neonatal care so that perspectives are not lost. Technology is not a god to be worshipped — only a tool to be harnessed for the greater good. The biological events and problems of the new-born period must be seen as an integral part of the whole of growth and development of the human with horizons which disappear backwards in time and forwards into the mists of future uncertainties.

10

The Management of "Medical Trivia" in Children: The Doctors' (New) Dilemma?

The Hong Kong Practitioner, 1985; 7:1,390–93

"We are trapped in social relations developed from centuries of self deception by both care givers and care receivers ...."

"Now medicine is real, expensive, potentially destructive, and absolutely demands discriminate use. But we retain social forms that make this difficult or impossible ...."
By a student (*Lancet*, 1983; 2:1,132–33)

Summary

The treatment of trivial paediatric medical problems has emerged as a new doctors' dilemma. Unrealistic parental expectations of their children's health together with uncritical and poorly informed medical practice is largely to blame. A radical rethink of the problem — which never appears in any "Recent Advances" series — is long overdue. This chapter defines the dilemma, its origins, manifestations and makes some suggestions (perhaps somewhat controversial) to resolve this issue.

The Dilemma

Setting the Scene

Many clinical problems for which children are brought by their parents to see doctors in out-patient clinics, accident and emergency units, general practice, and maternal and child health clinics are often medically trivial, resolving in time on their own accord. Fevers, coughs, headaches, sore throats and colds, abdominal pain, loose stools and feeding problems in babies provide the commonest examples. Yet, children must emerge out of a state of immunological virginity at birth. Is it therefore really surprising that respiratory tract infections, disorders due most often to viruses, are so common in childhood? They can be regarded almost as part of the normal growing up process — milestones to be passed! The gastrointestinal tract at birth is in a state of excited anticipation to cope with newly expected digestive demands in the early months after birth. Minor problems of adjustment will therefore inevitably arise.

Whilst in no way detracting from the unpleasantness of some of these problems to children, and their source of worry for parents, rarely are they life-threatening.

Parental Expectations

As the number of children in a family decreases, parental expectations for the attainment of optimum health in their children will increase — often to an unreasonable and unrealistic degree. These parents will often have more time to lavish concern on their children. Thus a child fifth in a family of seven who has a cough is less likely to cause as much concern to the mother as the second child in a family of two, simply because the mother has less time to be concerned.

In Hong Kong, for complex social and economic reasons, many infants and young children have to be looked after in the daytime by child-minders — relatives (often grandparents), amahs, etc. If these child-minders have occasion to take a child to see a doctor for one or other of these earlier mentioned trivial complaints, and emerge without "suitable medication," then the parents, on returning home in the evening, tired and wishing to see a nice healthy child, will often feel that the child-minder has not been living up to their responsibility. Furthermore, many of these guardians have themselves been brought up acknowledging the necessity for medical treatment for all complaints, however trivial; many parents have similar attitudes. For all these, and many other reasons, there is therefore considerable pressure on doctors at the primary care interface (whether this be in hospital, community clinic or office) to always exercise the therapeutic option of prescribing medication(s) in order to achieve an instant result. The demands made on all of us are often unreasonable. Indeed, it is all the more remarkable that these problems exist at a time when children's general health has never been better, through improved antenatal and perinatal care, widespread immunization against communicable diseases, good nutrition, improved housing and provision of better social and medical amenities.

The following dilemma therefore emerges: how can parental expectations of an unrealistic ideal for health in their children be dealt with by doctors, the majority of whom have a compulsive desire to prescribe medication for conditions many of which are trivial and which will, allowing Nature to take her course, resolve on their own accord?

Coping with the Problem

Can we deal satisfactorily with this problem? I often have nagging doubts.

A Compulsive Urge to Prescribe

In the first place, much undergraduate (and also continuing postgraduate) education is (in spite of greater awareness by clinical teachers in recent years) still largely irrelevant to a sizeable part of primary health care practice. All too little attention in so many disease-orientated paediatric curricula is given to understanding the common problems of childhood as those of a constantly changing, growing and developing organism that has to adjust and adapt itself to new environmental experiences. These common problems are too often considered simply as isolated episodes of illness without regard to the normal developmental biology of childhood. Secondly, the public are (often through no fault of their own) poorly informed about these problems. In general (and this is a universal not a local fault) they have a totally unreasonable expectation not only of what doctors are able to do but also about what "growing up" is all about in regard to its trials and medical tribulations. (What an appalling waste of all the potentially valuable years of school education?) The mystique of medicine and its apparent curative omnipotence mesmerizes parents and therefore indirectly their children.

As a direct consequence of these two complementary issues — parents who expect specific treatment and inadequately prepared doctors who (often misguidedly) wish to treat — antibiotics (often new and costly) are hurled around with gay abandon, and also cough medicines, decongestants, antiemetics, bowel sedatives to slow peristalsis, soy protein milk formulae and milk thickeners prescribed by the litre, in most instances without any labelling to provide their identity. Even more horrifying are hybrid mixtures of antipyretics and steroids to achieve instant lowering of temperature. But the problem does not stop there. If these children have occasion to be admitted to hospital, similar uncritical practices all too often abound, with over-investigation and inappropriately excessive treatments prescribed. This type of practice can best be described as mutually deceptive witchcraft.

Yet, and herein lies the main dilemma, if we as doctors do not live up to these expectations which parents have of us and prescribe medicine for an instant cure, then parents become dissatisfied and "shop around" until the "right medicine" is given by an apparently better informed doctor — often at considerable cost to themselves and potential harm to their children. This attitude is found not only in parents without benefit of an education, but also regrettably in those who have been thoroughly educated. No sector of society is immune.

Payment

In countries such as the United Kingdom where a doctor's salary is largely independent of the number of patients' seen, it is possible to practise medicine following the basic principles of clinical science (if these have been correctly taught). Yet the abuse of over-treatment of trivial ailments still abounds in that country for reason similar to those identified above. In Hong Kong and other countries where there is a sizeable private sector, the predicament is more complex and harder to resolve. In government and government-subvented sectors where doctors' salaries are not dictated by the standard and quality of their practice nor expectations of patients, sensible medical practice should still be possible. In private practice, however, there are imposed far greater distorting constraints on clinical practice. Thus, if a private practitioner simply tells parents not to worry (an often time-consuming exercise with 40 to 80 patients to be seen that morning), that the cough will get better in a few days, and that there is no need for specific treatment, the parents might well not accept the explanation, having been so deluded into believing in the power and mystique of medicine, and call "next door" where some treatment, often homeopathic in dosage, often harmful in effect, might be given largely to satisfy their expectations. Because most conditions which I have mentioned will improve on their own accord, the second doctor might therefore stand to suffer — his reputation will fall as also might his salary!

Yet the ancient Greeks divided their healers into three categories — the "knife" doctor; "herb" doctor and the "word" doctor. The latter in our technologically orientated society seems to have been lost by the wayside. Of course, many will say, often with justification, that the doctor is so swamped in a morass of vast numbers of patients that there is no time to talk — quicker to prescribe. Talking to parents is a luxury given to those who can arrange (at no lost cost to themselves) to see fewer patients. There is no denying much of the truth in this grumble and in seeking a solution to the problem, particular regard must be given to this consideration.

Dubious Drug Remedies

There must be a fundamental rethink about much of the drug prescription that currently exists. The number of medicaments currently available for the management of inconsequential illness are legion. Yet how many of these have really been adequately evaluated in clinical practice? Do cough medicines really work (the doses prescribed are often inadequate): in young children they are as likely to be dribbled onto their clothes as they are to enter the stomach! Indeed should a cough — Nature's expectorant — always be suppressed by drugs? Many decongestants we now know are potentially harmful, causing among other effects nightmares and hallucinations. Do they really work? Should they be given? Do the symptoms, often very trivial, really justify such attempted remedies? Antibiotics given for simple upper respiratory tract infections are usually inappropriate: frightening emerging patterns of drug resistance attest to such abuse. Drugs given to children with mild diarrhoea simply to delay intestinal transit time are of particularly dubious benefit. Is it really logical to delay transit time when increased peristalsis might be viewed as Nature's purgative to eliminate noxious substances? Many antiemetics prescribed can cause extrapyramidal side-effects. Milk "thickeners" for posseting are highly unphysiological. Likewise for abdominal pain — a complaint for which about 12% of children will at some time seek medical advice — antispasmodics are of no value. Yet all these medicines, both singly and in appalling combinations, are prescribed all over the world, rampantly and uncritically with apparent little regard either for the patients true well-being or to financial considerations of family or state providers of health.

The Solution

The management of "medical trivia" is one of the many challenges in paediatric practice (and also I am sure in adult medicine). Whether to treat or to leave alone often demands fine clinical judgement. Yet this subject never features in any "Recent Advances" series. It is an especially difficult problem to solve since what is required is a change in *attitude* on the part of both doctor and public (in this instance, the parents). Some of us in pessimistic mood may take the view that so entrenched are these attitudes on both sides of the equation that it will be impossible to overcome the inertia. In the short time that I have been working in Hong Kong, I have to admit to my attitude already having softened on occasions — cough linctuses, being prescribed where previously I would have withstood pressures to do so! (Perhaps at this juncture I should admit to having some experience in general practice in South Wales many years ago so that I am at least aware of what it is like to be on the other side of the desk and out of my ivory tower!)

Why therefore bother? Because if we do not, the practice of clinical medicine becomes relegated to a sloppy, pseudo-clinical science with the potential to cause more harm than good. Is this really what five years of a university medical education built on the foundation of ten years or so of schooling has done for most of us? Most medical students now passing through their undergraduate careers must be made aware of these controversies, as they are of the glamour of transplantation, *in vitro* fertilization, intensive care etc. With more realistic preparation, they might be better able to cope in the future than we are currently doing.

The other approach, a complementary one, is to tackle at the same time the other side of the coin — namely the misplaced expectations of parents. We should be taking far more opportunity to educate and counsel people about real expectations in health care. We should as doctors remove more of the mystique attached to medicine. Sympathy should not have as its invariable *sequitur*, medication. There exists an ideal opportunity in antenatal classes which about 99% of women attend. Might we perhaps not take greater opportunity during the preparation for childbirth in the many long hours of waiting in antenatal clinics, to help mothers understand more about problems they might expect in their children and methods by which these be managed? Such topics should of course also be introduced even earlier in schools, in courses of human biology — but with paediatricians actively involved. Such education should not be the sole prerogative of teachers.

Finally, why do parents so often not accept the judgement that a doctor might not consider treatment of a particular ailment to be justified? Are there seeds of mutual distrust between doctor and patient? Does this reflect our failure to be able to communicate with our patients and to show them appropriate empathy? With better-informed parents who accept and trust more, the clinics and waiting room should become less crowded, allowing the doctor more time to spend with real problems.

Unless a solution is sought to the therapeutic dilemmas posed by "trivial problems," the practice of much paediatric medicine will continue to diverge even further from its scientific roots. A break in the vicious circle is needed — but how and by whom? Perhaps the desire for and the need to prescribe the knife or herb is so deeply engrained in Man's subconscious spirit that it will never be removed.

I have made some suggestions. Do you have any more?

11

Bedwetting in Hong Kong Chinese Children: A Relatively Uncommon Problem

The Hong Kong Journal of Paediatrics, 1988; 5:65–66

Introduction

It is my impression that bedwetting at night (nocturnal enuresis) is a problem much less often encountered in hospital paediatric out-patient practice in Hong Kong than in the United Kingdom. To validate this impression, opportunity was taken in the course of a survey into the growth of normal children attending kindergartens and primary schools in one of Hong Kong's new towns to investigate when Chinese children stop wetting their beds at night.

Methods

Included in a questionnaire sent to the parents of about 2,500 children aged 3–7 years who were attending six normal kindergartens and the first class of a primary school in Sha Tin was the following question: "At what age did your child stop wetting the bed at night?" A total of 2,118 replies were obtained. From these the percentages of children reported to have stopped wetting their beds at 3, 5 and 7 years were determined.

Results and Comment

84%, 98% and virtually 100% of children were reported by their parents to be dry at 3, 5 and 7 years respectively. Using a questionnaire to obtain the information, there was no opportunity for further clarification of the answers as to the precise definition of being dry at night. I have interpreted the response as "socially meaningful" dryness at night; i.e. although occasional wet nights might be experienced, these were insufficient to alter the parents perception of dryness.

The reported incidence of bedwetting in Caucasian children varies widely. Meaningful comparison between studies is also made difficult since substantial methodological differences exist in respect to selection criteria, numbers of children studied, definitions, presentation and analysis of data, etc. With these reservations in mind, I have nevertheless made an attempt to obtain "average" values for dryness at night among Caucasian children. From multiple data published between 1956 and 1969 of the prevalence of nocturnal enuresis at various ages in Britain, Western Europe, North America and Australia, 68%, 84% and 89% of children at 3, 5 and 7 years of age were an average dry by night.[1] From these comparisons, Chinese children appear therefore to acquire bladder control at night at an earlier age.

But why? Might it be the result of an accelerated maturation of neurological mechanisms required to achieve nocturnal bladder continence? Could some socio-cultural factors such as early "training" by their mothers be operating? Whatever the explanation, and further study is warranted, the findings of this study go some way to explain the relative infrequency of bedwetting as a clinical problem in Hong Kong Chinese children.

Acknowledgements

I am grateful to Mrs. L. Lo, Miss S. Lui and Dr. S. Leung for help in analysing the data; to the many teachers in the schools for so willingly coordinating the study; to the parents for so conscientiously responding to the questionnaire; to Miss F. Lau for preparing the manuscript.

Reference

1. De Jonge, G. A. Epidemiology of Enuresis: A Survey of the Literature. In Kolvin, I., MacKeith, R. C., and Meadow, S. R., eds., *Bladder Control and Enuresis.* Clinics in Developmental Medicine, Nos. 48/49. London: Spastics International Medical Publications, William Heinemann Medical Books Ltd., 1973; 39–46.

12

Cot Death: How Common Is It in Hong Kong?

The Hong Kong Journal of Paediatrics, 1986; 3:87–92

Introduction

Cot death, the sudden infant death syndrome (SIDS), is the term given to the sudden, unexpected death (almost always) during sleep of a previously well baby where thorough post-mortem examination fails to adequately explain its cause. It is the single most common cause of post-neonatal death in infancy in the United Kingdom and many other Western countries, with an overall average incidence of 2–3/1,000.[1] A recently published paper from Glasgow showed cot death to be responsible for nearly 50% of deaths in 1981–82 of Scottish babies after the 7th day of life to the end of the first year.[2] Against this background, it therefore came as some surprise to me a few years ago to discover that cot death was a topic rarely discussed (other than by those preparing for their postgraduate examinations!) in Hong Kong. Until this year, it did not appear as a separate cause of death in the annual statistics of the Medical and Health Department.

Its Incidence in Hong Kong

This intriguing omission prompted me to undertake in January 1985 a survey of senior paediatricians, pathologists and accident and emergency doctors of their understanding of the problem of cot death in Hong Kong. What emerged was a convincing and wholly unanimous view that not only cot death but also its closely related problem, near miss cot death, was indeed rare in Hong Kong.[3] Between 1980–84, only 15 cases were documented in the records of the public mortuaries (Dr. F. Ong: personal communication), giving an approximate incidence of cot death over that 5-year period of about 0.05/1,000, a remarkable and almost unbelievably low figure. Especially interesting in Dr. Ong's series was that it contained four European babies (a considerable over-representation). The current 1984–85 *Department Report*,[4] the first to include sudden unexpected death as a separate cause of death, recorded only 3 cases in 1984. Retrospectively presented data from 1980–84 yielded a total of 23 cases. With about 400,000 births taking place in Hong Kong over this period and, for the sake of argument, allowing an incidence similar to that found in Western countries, between 800 to 1,000 cot deaths might have taken place.

A baby found dead at home has to be taken to one of the two public mortuaries (either on Hong Kong Island or the Kowloon peninsular) after being brought initially to a hospital accident and emergency department by the parents for death certification. Secretive disposal of a body in a place with such a high density of population, I am advised, is well nigh impossible. Perhaps a few cases were "missed" but surely not in the order of several hundred. When cot death occurs, it appears almost always in the post-neonatal age group. If cot death is being mislabelled or masquerading as other "hidden" diagnoses, such as bronchopneumonia (as was the case in many other countries prior to its eventual recognition), or "other ill defined and unknown causes of morbidity and mortality" (ICD code 799),[5] post-neonatal mortality figures would numerically reflect this. But this is far from being the case. Post-neonatal mortality is very low in Hong Kong, only 2.7/1,000 in 1984–85 in a total infant mortality rate of 9.1.[4] Had cot death occurred with similar incidence as in Western countries, post-neonatal mortality would be between 4–6/1,000 — which curiously enough happens to be a commonly quoted figure for this latter statistic in many of these countries.

Why Such an Uncommon Occurrence?

The inescapable conclusion is therefore that cot death is indeed extremely rare in Hong Kong. It is intriguing also to discover that in the United States, cot death has been recorded as least common in "Asian populations."[6] But why? Or should the question be turned around the other way — why does cot death occur with such high incidence in Western countries? Discussions with paediatricians from other Southeast Asian countries inform me that there also cot death is considered to be rare.

To begin an attempt to answer this question, some key assumptions are needed. Mine will be that apnoea is the immediate pathophysiological mechanism causing death, a view now widely held in those countries where sudden infant death is a problem. What factors in Hong Kong children might have some influence on this terminal event? I propose that we think along two main lines — factors in the environment and those in the host.

Environmental Factors

All studies emerging out of Western countries highlight a social background of deprivation to cot death — a syndrome of the underprivileged, with stress, unemployment, youthful parents, low standards of infant care, maternal smoking, multiparity, less than satisfactory antenatal care, poor housing, low incidence of breast-feeding all somehow contributing a fertile soil in which the seeds of potential cot death can germinate. The winter months seem to be especially vulnerable.[1,7] In considering this environmental background, there must immediately be acknowledged real difficulties which invariably arise in making comparisons with countries of markedly contrasting lifestyles, socio-economic and climate conditions, social attitudes and customs. Notwithstanding, yet at the same time admitting these reservations, interesting and sometimes paradoxical findings emerge in Hong Kong.

The incidence of breast-feeding, for example, is extremely low. The living environment for the great majority of people here is one of extreme crowding, with average population densities among the highest in the world. Many thousands continue to live in conditions which would be considered unacceptable in many Western countries. Such a low incidence of breast-feeding together with overcrowded living conditions (with an almost inevitability of increased respiratory tract infections) might, with current ideas and theories,[7] set the scene to favour the occurrence of cot death. Might other social and environmental factors somehow "balance out" these high-risk factors? There is greater social stability here with fewer very young marriages and unwanted babies and a stronger supporting extended family unit. Smoking is very uncommon, unemployment low and the overall standard of infant and antenatal care excellent. The winter months are also far less cold.

Might there even be some benefits to high-density living conditions. Babies are left alone much less. Sleep patterns could be different, thereby effecting subtle modulations to physiological responses concerned with ventilatory control. There is (virtually) never the question raised: "When can I put baby into his own room?" — an important early milestone in the lives of many young babies in Western countries. Might overall closer contact with the sleeping baby somehow lessen the risks of sudden death? Does a stronger extended family unit lessen the chances of filicide (child homicide by either parent) that, as has been recently been suggested, might account for between 2% and 10% of cot deaths?[8] Much speculation — regrettably no answers!

Factors in the Host

In my model, these revolve around the problem of apnoea, the likely immediate mechanism causing sudden death. For clinical convenience, cessation of breathing can be considered as of two chief aetiological types:[9] (1) central apnoea, where there is cessation of breathing movements due to lack of inspiratory drive from causes lying within the central nervous system; and (2) obstructive apnoea, in which air flow ceases with some continuing respiratory movements. Combinations of the two can also exist.

Let us consider first central apnoea. Its most prominent and frequently discussed association is with the recurrent and often prolonged apnoea of prematurely born babies. It is understandable therefore that these babies have become a prime focus of attention in any quest for the aetiology of cot death. The matter is, however, far from resolved.[10] That preterm babies and others admitted to a neonatal unit are more at risk of sudden and unexpected death has been well documented.[1,11,12] But whether this is due to central apnoea or other medical, social or environmental factors associated with prematurity remains to be determined. The incidence of infants weighing less than 1.5 kg at birth (most of whom would be born very prematurely) is reported to be much lower in Chinese than European populations.[13,14] Epidemiological comparisons of birth-weight categories between countries with diverse methods of data collection and analysis are, it has to be admitted, fraught with pitfalls and difficulties in interpretation. Nonetheless the purported lower incidence of extremely preterm babies might contribute to the lower incidence of cot death in Hong Kong — whatever its link with preterm birth.

Obstructive apnoea caused by interference with air flow in the upper respiratory passages has been implicated in the aetiology of cot death. Even mild upper respiratory tract symptoms of cough and rhinitis can accentuate periodic breathing and prolong apnoea in young infants.[15] Increasing upper airways resistance in new-born and young infants by occluding the nostrils reduces respiratory rate and ventilation volume.[16,17] The inappropriate ventilatory responses to upper nasal obstruction might arise in the course of a respiratory tract infection and therefore give some substance and credibility to the widely held view that respiratory symptoms are possibly causal to cot death.[7,18] But, and herein lies yet another paradox for Hong Kong, respiratory illnesses abound in infancy and childhood. If these truly play a major role in cot death, would not our babies also succumb? Certainly no miracle cures exist here for these extremely common paediatric problems.

There is one other aspect of obstructive apnoea which I currently find particularly intriguing, namely its causation by *external* obstruction of the airways. Wayte has recently drawn attention to smothering and suffocation leading to terminal asphyxia[19] as a possible final pathway to death (a view which does not seem to have been met with enthusiasm). Babies who lie *prone*, a not uncommon practice for nursing babies in Western countries, might be expected to more easily obstruct their airways, either by squashing the nostrils, the consequences of which would be worsened in the presence of upper airways congestion from infection, or even immersing the nose and mouth in vomit should it occur (a commonly reported terminal finding in cot death), thereby suffocating. A recent visitor to Hong Kong from the Institute of Child Health in London, Dr. John Pincott (Senior Lecturer in Histropathology), in a lecture at the Prince of Wales Hospital in November 1985, gave some interesting findings in 109 babies whom he had autopsied for cot death: 50% were found lying on their abdomen (25% face down, 25% face to side), 46% on the side and, most interesting, only 4% on the back. The tradition in Hong Kong, as indeed in many other parts of Southeast Asia and Japan, is for babies to be placed supine in the bed *for fear of suffocation* were they to lie prone. How provoking therefore a statement in a leading article in the *British Medical Journal* in 1971: “If death comes from failure to cope with respiratory difficulty it seems sensible to put a baby to sleep on his side or back rather than face down, when the weight of the trunk and not merely that of ribs and abdominal wall have to be lifted at each breath."[20]

Conclusion

These views I have put forward to explain the remarkable infrequency of cot death in Hong Kong compared with many Western countries are personal and unashamedly speculative. But perhaps no more so than the many speculations that continue to emerge at regular intervals out of the journals! There is little scientific basis for their credibility. They are offered more to catalyse thoughts and discussion on the problem than to provide a definitive explanation. I do wonder however whether lifestyle and "caretaking" practices are being underestimated in their possible influence on cot death in preference to more exotic explanations that regularly emerge.

All available data on the subject of cot death in Hong Kong are retrospective. Prospective study is necessary to identify the problem more precisely and to determine any possible aetiology. Such an investigation is currently being undertaken as a joint project between the Departments of Paediatrics and Community Medicine at The Chinese University of Hong Kong and the Department of Pathology of the University of Hong Kong. A better understanding of the problem as it exists might even contribute to a lessening of its occurrence in those countries where it continues as such an important cause of infant mortality.

Acknowledgements

I extend my thanks to the many paediatric, casualty, pathology and forensic colleagues who have helped me in preparing this chapter. Thanks and appreciation also to Miss J. Lee for preparing the manuscript.

References

1. Kelly, D. H., and Shannon, D. C. Sudden Infant Death Syndrome and Near Sudden Infant Death Syndrome. A Review of the Literature 1964 to 1982. *Pediatr Clin N Amer*, 1982; 29:1,241–61.
2. Arneil, G. C., Brooke, H., Gibson, A.A.M., *et al.* National Post-perinatal Infant Mortality and Cot Death Study. Scotland 1981–82. *Lancet*, 1985; 1:740–43.

3. Davies, D. P. Cot Death in Hong Kong: A Rare Problem. *Lancet*, 1985; 2:1,346–48.
4. *Department Report 1984–85*. Hong Kong: Medical and Health Department.
5. *WHO International Classification of Diseases*, 9th Revision, 1977.
6. Kraus, J. F., and Borhani, N. O. Post-neonatal Sudden Unexplained Death in California — A Cohort Study. *Am J Hygiene*, 1972; 94:497–99.
7. Knowwelden, J., Keeling, J., and Nicholl, J. P. *A Multicentre Study of Post-neonatal Mortality*. Sheffield: Medical Care Research Unit, University of Sheffield, 1984.
8. Emery, J. L. Infanticide, Filicide and Cot Death. *Arch Dis Child*, 1985; 60:505–7.
9. Apnoea Monitors and Sudden Infant Death. Report from the Foundation for the Study of Infant Death and the British Paediatric Respiratory Group. *Arch Dis Child*, 1985; 60:76–80.
10. Avery, M. E., and Frantz, I. D. To Breathe or Not to Breathe. What Have We Learned about Apnoeic Spells and Sudden Infant Death. *N Engl J Med*, 1983; 309:107–9.
11. Hillman, L., Hoffman, H. J., Jones, M., *et al.* Relationship of Prenatal and Natal Factors to SIDS: Preliminary Results of the NIHCH Cooperative Epidemiological Study of Sudden Infant Death Syndrome (SIDS) Risk Factors (Abstr). *Pediatr Res*, 1982; 16:291.
12. Brown, E. R., and Purohit, D. M. Sudden Death among Infants with Bronchopulmonary Dysplasia after Discharge from the Neonatal Intensive Care Unit. *Pediatr Res*, 1983; 18:305A.
13. Lau, S. P., Au-Yeung, C. L., Yeung, B.W.Y., *et al.* Major Determinants of Neonatal Mortality in Hong Kong. *H K J Paediatr*, 1984; 1:21–29.
14. Chalmers, I. Shanghai. *Lancet*, 1980; 1:137–39.
15. Bruhn, F. W., Mokrohisky, M. D., and McIntosh, K. Apnoea Associated with Respiratory Syncytial Virus Infection in Young Infants. *J Pediatr*, 1977; 90:382–86.
16. Swift, P.G.F., and Emery, J. L. Clinical Observations in Response to Nasal Occlusion in Infancy. *Arch Dis Child*, 1973; 48:947–51.
17. Purcell, M. Response in the Newborn to Raised Upper Airway Resistance. *Arch Dis Child*, 1976; 51:602–7.
18. Carpenter, R. G., Gardner, A., Jepson, M., *et al.* Prevention of Unexpected Infant Death. Evaluation of the First Seven Years of the Sheffield Intervention Programme. *Lancet*, 1983; 1:724–28.
19. Wayte, D. M. Smothering, Suffocation and Cot Deaths. *Lancet*, 1985; 1:114.
20. Cot Death (editorial). *BMJ*, 1971; 3:250–51.

13

Experiences with Mentally Handicapped Children in Pinehill Village

The Hong Kong Journal of Paediatrics, 1985; 2:76–80

It should go without saying that it is as important for children who are mentally handicapped to enjoy optimum physical health as it is for all other children. This assertion might seem a somewhat trite and even naive expression of the obvious but it must continue to be firmly stated since it is a philosophy which regrettably is all too often forgotten. These children must live to the full and benefit from whatever educational facilities are considered appropriate to their needs. What is so sad is that in addition to their chronic mental disability, many of them are all too often afflicted by other medical problems, many which they share with other children. Indeed, they are often more susceptible to general illnesses by virtue of their institutionalized environment, difficulties with personal hygiene and, in the case of children with Down's Syndrome, an intrinsic vulnerability to infection.

In many industrialized countries, the medical care of mentally handicapped children in special schools is usually the responsibility of community paediatricians working closely with the hospital services: general practitioners will sometimes provide this service. In parts of the world where paediatric community services have yet to be comprehensively developed, and I include Hong Kong in this category, alternative arrangements to look after the physical well-being of these children must evolve.

Pinehill Village

For nearly two years, I have had the privilege to serve the Pinehill Village Schools as honorary paediatrician. This Village in Tai Po is operated by the Hong Kong Association for the Mentally Handicapped and is partly government-subvented. Its aims are to help all mentally handicapped children develop their potential to the full. There are five projects in the Village: Pinehill Village Pre-school Centre (weekly and complete residential) for mildly and moderately mentally handicapped children aged 3–6 years; Pinehill Village School (a day school) for the moderately mentally handicapped children aged 6–16 years; Pinehill Village No. 2 School (a weekly residential school) for severely mentally handicapped children aged 6–16 years; Pinehill Village No. 3 School (a complete residential school) for severely mentally handicapped children aged 6–16 years; and Pinehill Village Advanced Training Centre aimed at providing vocational training for mildly or moderately mentally handicapped youths aged 16–20 years.

Causes of Handicap

The aetiologies of handicap in these children are many and varied. Down's Syndrome inevitably contributes a sizeable proportion. Complications of encephalitis and meningitis and seizures in early childhood present along with a variety of rare syndromes such as Hunter's Syndrome, tuberous sclerosis and unusual chromosome anomalies. There are a few children suffering the consequences of very delayed diagnosis of congenital hypothyroidism. However, what I have been surprised to find is that so many children have no apparent cause for their chronic mental disability. Are these simply the extreme end of the normal distribution for mental ability? Are many the consequences of adverse social and other environmental influences? The extent of our medical ignorance in the area of mental handicap is all too often exposed in our failure to understand its aetiology. Without this much of our treatment is so empirical as to be almost meaningless. There is endless scope for research.

Possibly the most distressing children in the Village are orphans who have been labelled "mentally handicapped" not for any obvious physical reason but more as a consequence of lack of stimulation and behavioural disturbance through their own emotional conflicts during their passages through various orphanages and other institutions. I strongly take issue with the use of the term "mental handicap" for most of these children. Disturbed they might be, underachieving their potential they undoubtedly are: mentally handicapped they are surely not. This is a devastating term to use; all chances of later adoption and even appropriate educational placement being rendered extremely difficult. As doctors we need to be far more aware of the drastic consequences which can result from dangling labels of loosely meaning diagnoses (often inaccurate) around children's necks. Once placed they can rarely be removed. They resemble tattoo marks. To see these children with brains capable of normal function spending most of their days and nights with children who are mentally handicapped is a disturbing experience and one which should catalyse greater efforts to resolve the problem. The longer they mix with these children, the more will they take on their mannerisms and abnormal behavioural traits. But how aware is our high technology-orientated community of the existence of these children? Sadly, not very!

Medical Commitment

Attending Pinehill continues to be a valuable and rewarding experience, teaching me not only about the spectrum of, and the approach to, mental handicap in Hong Kong (including particularly educational aspects about which I know very little), but also the many and varied medical problems which can afflict these children in their daily lives. It is also a pleasure to work alongside so many people who carry out a job which so many would seem to contain so little job satisfaction: far less glamorous than hospital work yet, in many respects, more demanding. So often the concern of paediatricians such as myself when we practise in a general capacity is with the principal handicapping problem. There is, somewhat ashamedly to admit, all too little awareness of the children's general medical problems which, if left unattended, can so seriously interfere with their well-being and education. This in turn will add further problems to themselves as well as to their already stressed families.

I hold a "surgery" every Wednesday morning in the Village, assisted by the nursing and teaching staff of the school, when a miscellany of problems are seen: epilepsy; communicable diseases (particularly diarrhoea); fevers, scabies and skin infections; worms, respiratory tract infections; ear infections (which are particularly common); cardiac problems in children with Down's Syndrome; in some instances terminal care, etc. All children admitted to the school are given a thorough examination (in addition to the compulsory routine stool, urine and chest X-ray insisted upon by the Association). When the time comes for their discharge, a final clinical examination is given, a problem list completed and a letter of referral or transfer given to their families to facilitate any transition of care which has to take place. While they are attending the school, parents are given a health record sheet which includes their children's current condition and any medication. This enables the parents to communicate more effectively about their children's medical condition if they need to seek medical advice in other hospitals over holidays or weekends. It also allows hospitals to provide better care for the children since attending paediatricians will be in possession of up-to-date information about the children's problems.

My association with Pinehill Village has made me reach the conclusion (which of course may not be shared by others) that perhaps one approach in Hong Kong to providing regular, suitable and consistent medical support for our mentally handicapped children in schools and other related institutions (orphanages etc.) is for paediatricians to extend their services beyond their hospital and office bases and visit these community schools on a regular basis. This approach is already being implemented by some paediatricians elsewhere in the territory. The well-worn comment of "too little time" is too often an excuse and not an adequate enough reason for not providing such a service. It is surely right for us as paediatricians to try to organize our departments and ourselves to help some of the more vulnerable members of our paediatric community, even if this does mean an added commitment to an already busy timetable.

The regular weekly commitment that I have described provides consistency and continuity of care, far more so I believe than the occasional brief consultation on an irregular basis: it is better to regularly anticipate that problems will occur rather than wait to be called. Policies for certain common medical problems can be better worked out and implemented with the teaching and nursing staff, as for example the management of children with convulsions, domestic accidents and gastroenteritis. Talks can be given to staff to help them understand some of the frequently encountered medical problems and their basic management. I am under no illusion that the medical care which is provided is better than that given by any other hospital to which a child might be referred. But in having someone who attends regularly once a week, the nursing and teaching staff are often saved the worry of making a decision whether or not to refer elsewhere — in our case to the Jockey Club Clinic in Tai Po or other hospitals in Hong Kong.

Fewer taxis have to be ordered. The staff do not have to leave the school so often (this by itself is an appalling misuse of a valuable resource). The children are less disturbed. If problems arise between clinic days, these can be immediately referred either to myself or to other members of our department. With the opening of the Prince of Wales Hospital, it is now far easier for children to be admitted to hospital and looked after by doctors who know the children. Follow-up can be undertaken at the school, saving many unnecessary journeys to hospital out-patient clinics.

Teaching

The association between our department and Pinehill is now entering an exciting new phase. Each week we are sending two medical students who are in their second clinical year paediatric module. They spend two days living in the Village learning a little about the problems of living with and caring for mentally handicapped children. These visits are not intended to make the students learn all the physical signs and symptoms of handicap (so dearly loved by generations of students and teachers!). Instead they are intended more to provide them with a total experience of, and an insight into, the problems of mental handicap — especially the immense demands made on the children, their families and on those who have to care for them in special schools. They learn that with appropriate care children, however handicapped, will progress and live with dignity. Those who are mild to moderately retarded will, through the Advanced Training Centre, acquire vocational skills to give them the potential to make a valuable contribution to society. Our students sit in during classes and meal times; they help put the small children to bed and dress them in the mornings. They also attend the Wednesday surgery to learn about medical problems in these children. I must express my sincere appreciation and thanks to the Hong Kong Association for the Mentally Handicapped, and especially to all staff of the Village, for their enthusiasm, support and cooperation in this exciting new venture. They put themselves out considerably to make the students welcome. Having students regularly throughout the year is an added burden for an already stretched staff but we hope it will be worthwhile, helping to make a new generation of young doctors more aware of the needs of these disadvantaged children and those who care for them in the multiplicity of their problems.

Conclusion

As paediatricians we must be more aware of these "other children," the silent numbers all too often tucked away out of sight and out of mind for the convenience of society. We must recognize far more than we do our responsibilities to chronic disability and rehabilitation. I am concerned that even in our more enlightened age there is still an overemphasis on the developments of medical services in hospitals and too little awareness of the need to develop services concerned with chronically disabled children — especially teachers and nurses, psychologists, speech therapists, occupational therapists and physiotherapists etc. (The same argument applies equally to the chronically disabled adult.) The problem will not go away. We should take every opportunity to support (sympathetically and positively) these and many other workers in their activities and demands — that is, of course if as true paediatricians, we are concerned with the welfare of all children. Our medical role is often a small one — a small cog in an otherwise complex big wheel in which many others, professional and non-professional alike, play a more important role. In no way are most of us, in our capacity as general paediatricians, equipped to do much more than to diagnose the nature of handicap and to manage their medical problems. Yet if we accept this role and apply ourselves to ensure that these children enjoy the best possible physical health, then we are making an important contribution to their families' happiness, well-being and dignity.

14

Medical Responsibilities to the Mentally Handicapped[*]

The Hong Kong Practitioner, 1987; 9:2,687–96

"The mentally retarded person has a right to economic security and to a decent standard of living. He has the right to perform productive work, or to engage in any other meaningful occupation to the fullest possible extent of his capabilities."

U.N. Declaration on the Rights of the Mentally Handicapped 1971

Introduction

As the environmental scourges of malnutrition and serious infectious disease in children have been progressively eradicated from our community over the past few decades, a major area of paediatric concern to have emerged is that of neuro-developmental disability affecting the brain, mind, body and special senses, singly, or more commonly, in combination. The major contributor to these problems is mental handicap.

This chapter deals with the nature of mental handicap and the responsibilities of doctors in general to those so affected, particularly children. The major theme is intended as a rhetorical question, asking whether as doctors (in both community and hospital) we have satisfactorily defined our role in this exceedingly complex world of multi-disciplinary interaction that is mental handicap. Anticipating some of my conclusions I have to

* Based on a lecture given to the Zonta Club of Hong Kong, 30 April 1986.

admit with some regret that in Hong Kong, as in many other parts of the world, attitudes to, and the medical care of, the mentally handicapped continue to lag considerably behind those concerned with the management of acute physical illness. For too long have the mentally handicapped been allowed to remain out of both sight and mind. The relative neglect of their problems in comparison with those of the more glamorous and immediately rewarding areas of medical care in both undergraduate and postgraduate curricula embarrassingly attests to this. There is however reason now for greater optimism as health professionals, educationalists, government authorities and the public at large seem to have grown more aware of the needs of these disadvantaged people who, when looked after with care, kindness and sympathy they deserve, can contribute so much to society. Our ultimate duty to them must be to ensure that they, with their families, enjoy their deserved dignity and respect and an opportunity to contribute and integrate as much as possible in our community.

The Nature of Mental Handicap

There is no universally accepted definition of mental handicap.** For the purposes of this chapter, I define it as a disability of thought, reasoning and memory leading to a limited ability to acquire that most vital of human attitudes, adaptation to the routine demands of day-to-day living originating in childhood and due either to: (1) abnormal development of the brain early in its ontogeny (organic mental retardation); or (2) the expression of one tail of the normal Gaussian curve for intelligence (familial mental retardation). At the outset mental handicap has to be clearly distinguished from mental disorder. At the risk of oversimplification, mental disorder implies more a state of disturbed behaviour in a mind housed usually within a normally

** The Warnock Report in 1978 recommended the term "children with learning difficulties" for children given the diagnosis of mental handicap or educationally subnormal. The learning difficulties in turn were further categorized as "mild," "moderate" and "severe." Although in Special Education establishments this concept has been accepted and applied, in general parlance the term "mental handicap" has been retained. However providing it is used and applied correctly, the term "mentally handicapped" need not be to the detriment of affected children.

developed brain, in contrast to mental handicap which is more a state of arrested or incomplete development of higher mental functioning. Failure to appreciate these differences regularly leads to misconceptions of such a magnitude as to often seriously interfere with social progress required for the management of these increasingly important problems.

The special educational needs of mentally handicapped children have to be provided by methods and means which differ from those available to children of normal intelligence, either in special schools or in integrated projects in normal schools, in order to help them develop to the full their mental potential. As adults the mentally handicapped need, to varying extents depending on the severity of handicap, continued and lifelong shelter because of inability to adequately look after themselves.

Mental handicap in Hong Kong is traditionally considered in three tiers — severe, moderate and mild according to the measured Intelligence Quotient (I.Q.):

1. Severe: I.Q. < 25 — These children are usually unable to benefit from vocational training and are wholly dependent on others for their handicap although often its exact aetiology will not be found.
2. Moderate: I.Q. 25–49 — Minimal language development can emerge in these children and with appropriate training, self-care skills and simple tasks can be achieved.
3. Mild: I.Q. 50–70 — Many children in this category will, with guidance and patience, be capable of developing social and communicative skills. With suitable training, they should be able to acquire appropriate social and vocational skills with comparatively little supervision. This category will of course include the tail of the normal distribution curve of ability where social and cultural factors play such an important role in determining the expression of intelligence. In such children, I prefer to use the term "slow learner" in preference to "mild grade mental handicap" for fear of irreversible stigmatization.

Placing an individual child into one of these three categories of mental handicap is necessary for educational placement, curriculum planning and designing training programmes. However, in assessing ability through I.Q. determination it must be appreciated that the initial assessment will not necessarily provide a true estimate of ability. Several years and continued assessment are usually needed to allow true potential to be ascertained.

Mental handicap of organic origin is often associated with other problems of neuro-developmental disability. The effective and compassionate care of the mentally handicapped — their learning disabilities, physical and behavioural problems and the community — will therefore often demand a collaborative multi-disciplinary approach with professionals of diverse skills working harmoniously with each other in order to achieve the best possible fulfilment of the disabled persons' potential — teachers trained in special educational methods, physiotherapists, occupational therapists, educational and clinical psychologists, psychiatrists, specialists in speech and language development, medical specialists (especially those involved in eye, ear and musculoskeletal disorders), nurses, paediatricians, neurologists, general practitioners, etc. Depending on the spectrum of disability will be the involvement of these people who will provide a complex (and often very confusing) mosaic of help, in roles that are physically and emotionally demanding, time-consuming and from the community viewpoint, costly.

Causes of Mental Handicap

A clinical/pathological model of mental handicap to facilitate understanding of its causes, associations and later management is shown in Figure 1. In its many and varied forms, mental handicap can be likened to a flower. The stem that immediately bears the "symptomatic flower" of handicap is the arrested or incomplete development of the brain. Because of the variety of possible development insults and their variable effects on the brain's many higher functions, together with the complexity of neural structures within the brain, this "flower" is often associated with smaller "offshoots"-associated problems — all of which can together be collectively termed the *spectrum of neuro-developmental handicap*. These include epilepsy, physical disorders such as cerebral palsy, behavioural problems, etc. The spectrum and interaction of these disabilities depend on those parts of the brain affected by, and the timing and nature of, the original insult. When we talk of children who are mentally handicapped, we are usually referring to this problem as the *major* neuro-developmental disability.

The pathophysiological stem emerges out of the complex "root system" of aetiologies, each figuratively having an independent access to the

Figure 1. Causes of Mental Handicap.

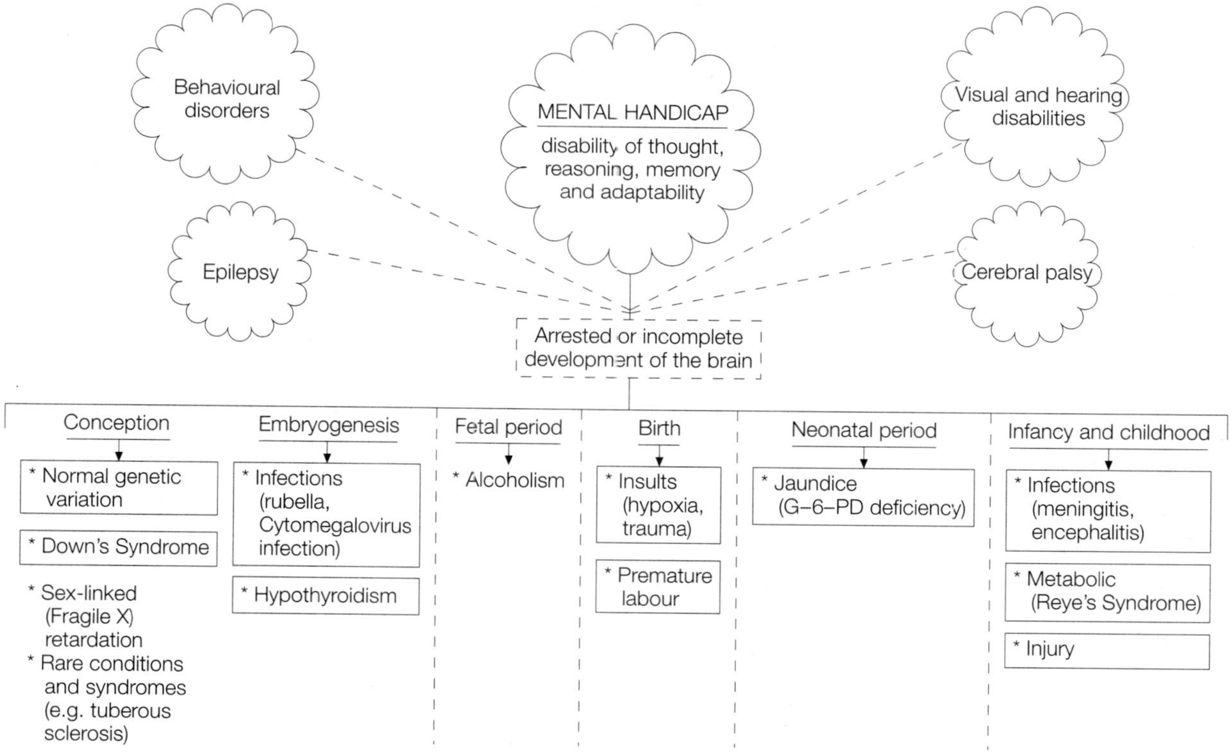

stem. These are best considered according to the stage of development reached when mental handicap is determined. For example:

Conception — genetic variation and Down's Syndrome
Embryogenesis — hypothyroidism, rubella virus infection
Fetal life — alcoholism
Birth — asphyxia
New-born period — jaundice
Childhood — meningitis, social/environmental influences

I have included social/environmental causes in this latter category somewhat reluctantly (in actual practice, there will also be to an indeterminate extent a contribution from the genotype) since to label children whose mental function is less than adequate because of environmental deprivation mentally handicapped is, I believe, both inaccurate and incorrect — the term "slow learner" being infinitely preferable, a point I shall return to later. Its inclusion here bows to local convention.

Consideration of this clinico-pathological model leads to a conclusion which is all too often neglected by doctors and all who are involved in the care of the mentally handicapped, that mental handicap is no more a diagnosis than is headache, abdominal pain, etc. It is simply a convenient label for a constellation of learning disabilities. The term mental handicap should never be used without being prepared to relate to its pathophysiology and aetiology. We must not dangle labels for our convenience around the necks of these children. To do so is to court disaster. Labels can rarely be removed and they can often confuse and be stigmatic. Furthermore, if mental handicap is to be considered a diagnosis in itself, there will subconsciously be less drive and commitment to ascertain its cause. Without full knowledge and awareness of this vital principle, management programmes become misapplied, an especially tragic circumstance if there is a potentially remediable cause for the handicap.

Incidence of Mental Handicap

In any population, the incidence of mental handicap will be determined by four main factors:

1. The incidence at conception, prenatal and postnatal life of abnormalities that can later lead to handicap.

2. Effects of individual and community attitudes towards termination of pregnancies for conditions that would otherwise lead to states of progressive disability.
3. Survival of affected babies after birth.
4. Methods and reliability of later ascertainment of the extent and severity of mental handicap.

The incidence of mental handicap appears to be fairly uniform in parts of the world where studies have been undertaken to determine its incidence. An approximate rate is 30 per 1,000 children and of these about 15% are severe grade, 40% moderate, 45% mild. Statements continue to appear in medical and general literature that in a large proportion of children the cause for handicap cannot be ascertained, but this is misleading and does not recognize several important recent studies in the field. In a group of severe grade children in Sweden, a definite aetiology was found in as high as 86%: 73% were regarded as being of prenatal origin, 10% perinatal and 3% developing after birth. In another comprehensive study from Salford (Britain) of 396 severely handicapped children born between 1961 and 1980, prenatal origins occurred in 55%, perinatal in 20% and postnatal in 10%. These accounted for 85% of all cases. Fewer studies of moderate/mild handicap have been made but from those available genetic-socio/cultural interactions play a very important role.

There are as yet no reliable data for the incidence of mental handicap in Hong Kong, but we have no reason to believe that there are significant deviations from other countries with a similar pattern of childhood morbidity and mortality. In time it would be hoped that an accurate estimate will emerge. Precise details are needed as a matter of urgency since without them it is impossible to allocate sufficient resources for the care of the mentally handicapped, both as children and adults.

Responsibilities of Doctors to the Mentally Handicapped

This overview of the nature, causes and incidence of mental handicap should allow the responsibilities of doctors in general to be better appreciated and understood. I propose these to be considered in four broad categories: prevention; early identification and assessment; continuing medical care; and advocacy and education.

Prevention

Our most important collective responsibility towards the problem of mental handicap must surely be towards its prevention. In this function, doctors of many disciplines must at some stage contribute. Some examples relevant to Hong Kong are considered here:

Prenatal Diagnosis

Amniocentesis does have the potential to diagnose and, through pregnancy termination, reduce the incidence of Down's Syndrome, the single most common cause of severe mental handicap. This method of secondary prevention is not, however, without its difficult moral and ethical quandaries, let alone the fact that of all children with mental handicap those with Down's Syndrome are often the easiest to look after, not being complicated by cerebral palsy, severe behavioural disturbances and other neuro-developmental problems so often found in other disabled children. (Children with Down's Syndrome will of course always require care and protection in the community but whether they deserve to be deprived of this by virtue of the simple possession of an additional chromosome is ethically contentious.) With time it is likely that other genetic sources of mental handicap will be available by prenatal diagnosis. Already one such example to emerge is the Fragile X Syndrome — a sex-linked disorder due to a fragile band q 27 on the X chromosome (affecting males and carried by females with an approximate incidence of 1:2,500) causing a moderate degree of intellectual handicap. Fragile X-linked mental retardation is now reputed to be the next most common cause of mental retardation in males after Down's Syndrome.

Genetic Counselling

The best example of this primary preventive approach is perhaps the general encouragement to mothers to have children when they are relatively young to lessen the likelihood of Down's Syndrome. Where there is a family history of previous mentally retardation strongly suggestive of a genetic aetiology, as for example tuberous sclerosis, genetic counselling is essential.

Good Perinatal Care

Though birth insults (hypoxia, trauma, haemorrhage) and premature birth are usually associated more with cerebral palsy and specific sensory handicaps, these environmental hazards are also a well-recognized cause of mental handicap when those parts of the brain to be later concerned with cognitive function are injured. Identification of high-risk pregnancies with delivery in a hospital appropriately equipped with both human and technological resources to manage perinatal disorders which can lead to irrecoverable mental handicap is an essential primary preventive measure.

Neonatal Metabolic Screening

Depending on the ethnic composition of a population under consideration will be the disorders requiring screening. In Hong Kong, the two principal disorders which can, unless detected early, lead to mental handicap are congenital hypothyroidism (about 1 per 3,500 live births) and glucose–6–phosphate dehydrogenase (G–6–PD) deficiency occurring in about 5% of males and 0.3% females and a potential cause of profound brain damage through kernicterus. By early replacement therapy with thyroxine in the former, and the avoidance of haemolytic stress in the latter, the brains of children with these disorders should develop normally.

Immunization against Rubella

This scheme was commenced in 1978 in Hong Kong and currently over 95% of teenage girls in schools are immunized. By preventing rubella embryopathy, in which microcephaly can so often be an integral part, an important contribution to preventing severe mental handicap is made.

Effective Treatment of Epileptic Fits, Meningitis, Encephalitis, etc.

How the incidence of mental handicap can be reduced by the prompt recognition, diagnosis and treatment of these disorders — methods of tertiary prevention — has yet to be determined. However, our special schools have many examples of children who, in their case records, are mentioned to have suffered previous fevers, fits and infections: though probably contributing only a small proportion of the total, rendering the best possible care for these conditions is something that we as doctors should be able to do and its importance never underestimated in minimizing later mental handicap.

Environment and Social Improvement

One vital area of prevention often overlooked, or never even thought of, concerns the care of children socially and emotionally deprived or abandoned by their families or brought up in very blunted emotional surroundings, thereby preventing achievement of their full mental potential. The parents of these children have themselves often been deprived, or because of financial need, have had to leave their children to the care of elderly relatives or other child-minders who are unable to provide the searching and stimulating environment needed by the inquisitive developing child. These socio-culturally deprived children can easily withdraw into themselves and in addition to becoming emotionally and physically stunted, can lag profoundly behind in their mental development. Although I am personally reluctant to label socially and emotionally deprived children as mentally handicapped, its present adoption in Hong Kong makes reference to this problem essential in the context of prevention. These children need to be considered more as slow learners than mentally handicapped.

Although not a primary medical responsibility, there is still a lot that we can do to help these children. By simply being aware of their existence and identifying the problem early on, much can be done to prevent the disturbing sequelae of deprivation. Thus, if in the initial assessment of children who are referred to us on account of slow development, we find the most likely cause to be in the child's social environment, this should be clearly stated and terms such as mental handicap avoided. (This is an example of what I have previously mentioned about not dangling around necks of children labels that cannot be withdrawn.) In recognizing social and other environmental origins, available community resources should then be mobilized to help these children. Appropriate educational placement, not alongside truly mental handicapped children, might offer a better future for them. One example of what can be achieved in this regard relates to an experience in one of our Special Schools for the mentally handicapped. Three children previously labelled as mentally handicapped succeeded, with much time being spent on their educational and social rehabilitation, in entering a normal kindergarten. Within six months, all three succeeded in having the label of mental retardation removed and this contributed significantly to their being accepted on the International Adoption Register. All three are now happy and established in adoptive families in the United States. There are sadly, however, all too many children here in Hong Kong who have been less fortunate and continue their education alongside mentally handicapped children, never thereby fulfilling their true potential, with a future shrouded in gloom and uncertainty.

Prevention of Accidents

Road traffic injuries, and accidents in the home may bring about injuries to the head which may result in permanent mental disability. As doctors, we should take every opportunity to remind parents of their responsibilities and to the public in general on road and other environmental safety precautions.

Early Identification and Assessment

After prevention, two closely interrelated areas must be considered the most important of medical responsibilities to the mentally handicapped — its early identification and full assessment. As doctors, we are very much in the front line when it comes to initial detection, suspicion leading to diagnosis being promoted by several situations:

1. In the course of routine assessments, maternal and child health clinics are as part of the Comprehensive Observation scheme and other developmental surveillance programmes. Suspicion of abnormal development leads to referral for further specialist management. What usually initiates concern about possible early mental handicap is a slowness in a child's psychomotor achievements although there must be admitted a real difficulty in often being unable to discriminate the abnormal from the biological tail of normality so early in development. Not to be aware of this will, on occasions, cause great hardship to the family and child concerned by over-diagnosing mental handicap.
2. At birth a pointer towards later mental disability can be made with certainty in certain conditions such as Down's Syndrome, and in some other very rare disorders of genetic or prenatal origin. Such early identification anticipates follow-up and suitable later referral and management.

3. Promoted by parental worry about failure of their baby to be developing normally.
4. In the course of following up in hospital clinics babies considered at high risk. These include babies born prematurely, requiring ventilation, suffering complications such as intraventricular haemorrhage, intra-partum asphyxia, etc.

Assessment of Handicap

As previously mentioned, the full diagnosis of mental handicap includes three distinct levels: (1) the disability itself; (2) the mechanism immediately responsible; and (3) its aetiology. Emerging out of this comprehensive diagnosis will be the full extent of neuro-developmental disability. But unfortunately in both medical and psychological reports, this rarely happens. Mental handicap is a term which is all too often considered in itself a diagnosis. In the early stages of problem identification and assessment, it is important, through careful and thorough history taking and examination, to explore the fullest possible extent of any other associated neuro-developmental disability — epilepsy, cerebral palsy, special sense disorders, learning problems, etc. — all these problems being offshoots and consequences of abnormal brain development. An impression of the impact of the disability on the child and its family must also be gained to provide some insight into the social resources needed to help in the day-to-day management on a practical level.

A full assessment will often need to take place at some stage in a Child Assessment Centre, fully equipped and staffed with personnel to investigate the child's physical, psychological and social development, such as the Arran Street Child Assessment Centre in Kowloon. There is a need for more such centres throughout the territory and it is encouraging to note that there are plans for a further six in Hong Kong. Let us hope that they will all truly materialize and not remain a figment of government drawing board imagination! There is a serious lack in Hong Kong of facilities for both the assessment and later management of mental handicap and its associated problems including educational placement. Contrast this with the greatly improved in-patient hospital services for children, many of whom have straightforward illnesses, easily managed and of short duration.

Having admitted to this need for a wider provision of assessment and management facilities, I would like at the same time to caution that paediatricians should not become over-reliant on the Assessment Centre. Just as secondary care paediatricians should be able to initially approach most problems (the special interest tertiary care paediatrician being valued for the problems requiring a more specialized knowledge), so also should adequately trained paediatricians be able to cope with most developmental problems in the early stages. There is a tendency for many doctors, once they "smell" a developmental problem, to hastily reach for their referral pad! Conceptually after all there is little difference in the clinical analysis of a developmental problem as one of a more physical nature. Also, in all major hospitals there are paediatricians, physiotherapists, occupational therapists, social workers, medical specialists (orthopaedic, ENT and ophthalmological surgeons), all of whom can be formed into a multi-disciplinary assessment and management team. Unfortunately, there is a serious dearth of psychologists and this provides a major impediment to assess special educational needs without which educational placement is often difficult. I believe that every encouragement must be given to hospitals to develop their own assessment management teams. These would help relieve the burden on the Assessment Centre, reduce long waiting lists and allow them in turn to act more in a tertiary care capacity to cope with particularly difficult problems. With so much of contemporary paediatrics concerned with developmental disorders, for paediatricians not to play a more dominant role in assessment and management is surely a waste of valuable trained resource.

Undoubtedly, one of the hardest tasks confronting the doctor with a disorder such as mental handicap for which no cure exists is to explain to the parents the diagnosis and outcome in terms easily understood. This is a skill that regrettably is all too often performed poorly, fascination in the disease process being more interesting than the human aspects of the problem. Often many visits will be needed to explain harsh realities to parents for whom the future will often look bleak. Doctors need to show much greater empathy. Communicative skills in this field are sadly lacking with all too many doctors being unable to know how to begin to talk to a mentally handicapped child and his/her parents. Wherever possible the same group of persons must see the parents and child on each occasion. Herein lies the strength of the hospital assessment team which must be developed alongside larger regional assessment units.

Continuing Medical Care

Once identification and full assessment have been made, the overall management programme of mentally handicapped children can be considered in three major areas.

Education

To help the child develop its abilities and potential to the full, special and integrated child care centres, special schools, and training centres all have a key role to play. In this the medical role is small and supportive and very much subordinate to educational aspects.

Social

To support the child and the family, ensuring that full advantage is taken of such social supporting facilities as the disability allowance and other financial and social entitlements, the medical role here is again supportive to social and other community workers.

Medical-associated Problems

Depending on the interest, available resources and the nature of the problem will be the part played by doctors in this area of responsibility. *But contribute all doctors must.* These medical problems can be considered in three main groups:

1. Problems linked directly with any primary brain pathology — Examples include epilepsy, hearing problems, cerebral palsy, hydrocephalus. Epilepsy deserves special mention as the most common major problem in the mentally handicapped. Often seizures are difficult to control. Fits are varied and usually complex. Drug compliance is variable, children having difficulty in taking medication and parents sometimes failing to recognize the importance of administering the drugs at home. There is a need for all these children to be seen regularly, and wherever possible by the same doctor, to maintain optimum continuing care. It is just not good enough to wait for the problem to develop. Continuing care of the mentally handicapped child with a medical problem is one that as a whole we doctors undertake very badly.

2. Related physical disabilities — For example heart disease in children with Down's Syndrome where shared hospital care is needed.
3. Day-to-day clinical problems — These constitute worries similar to those experiences by non-mentally handicapped persons. They include: (1) *Skin problems*, particularly septic spots, non-specific dermatoses, paronychia and ringworm, problems encountered especially in residential schools. They are often made worse through self-inflicted trauma from scratching, etc.; (2) *Ear discharge* caused by chronic otitis media and externa, is, if looked for, very common and the result probably of late and badly managed ear infections, a task made even harder by failure of the child to explain their symptoms. Examination of the ears of children in special homes and schools often makes a horrifying reality; (3) *Respiratory and gastrointestinal infections*, as in other children these are common. With scrupulous care given to personal hygiene and food preparation, risks of outbreaks of enteric infections can be minimized in special schools.

This commitment to the medical problems of the mentally handicapped is vital, but one which is all too often poorly undertaken. It does well to remind ourselves that it is the right of all children to enjoy optimum health. Unfortunately, mentally handicapped children often suffer unnecessarily the "inverse care" law. Without enjoying optimum physical health, disabled persons will never be able to fulfil their potential. We will not help the mentally handicapped enjoy health to the full by sitting in our hospital clinics and offices waiting for them to be brought to us with their problems. Those of you who have been into schools and other institutions for the handicapped will know the massive upheaval to take one child to a clinic or doctor. Teachers, nurses and helpers have to take time off — a dreadful waste of a valuable and limited resource. Taxis or buses have to be arranged. Hours are spent in accident and emergency departments and out-patient clinics. Even when children visit hospitals, there is often a reluctance to communicate to the school about outcome. There is a need to keep these children *out of hospital*, often a strange and frightening place for them. Doctors should be more committed and seek these children, not to simply await problems to reach them. It is encouraging that more and more paediatricians are now becoming attached to schools for purposes of improving the health and welfare of the children. Much, however, remains to be achieved. If we can better deal with their medical problems, mundane in terms of medical fascination though they might be, their lives would be made much happier.

Because of frequent multiplicity of their problems, mentally handicapped children, along with their parents, often spend many hours a week visiting different specialists. We should be offering better and more efficient general help to cope with the vast array of services which are made available but whose administrative complexities often defeat all but the stoutest of hearts! We do not on the whole perform these coordinating functions well — largely because of lack of knowledge, empathy and awareness — again a sign of the cocoon-like nature of our profession. The "system" for these families often seems (and indeed is) endlessly complicated and a continuing hurdle to overcome. If as doctors we concerned ourselves more with practical aspects of care, thinking a little more of the constant upheaval from hospital visits, we would do all a great favour. Waiting many hours in a clinic, often to be seen by an inexperienced doctor for a few minutes, to what avail? What to do if a wheelchair breaks down? How can a hearing aid be repaired or an ear mold replaced? How to ensure payment of disability allowance? etc.

Are all visits to clinics really important? Cannot they be better synchronized? The world of the family of a handicapped person is often an endless series of clinic visits with little to show for them at the end of the day, a form of perpetual motion with little to look forward to. This should be something which as doctors we can and should do something about if we are so motivated.

Advocacy and Education

Our final responsibility is that of advocacy to help promote awareness and a social conscience, drawing the public's attention to the plight of mentally handicapped people and their families. Many come from the poorer sectors of our community and are less able to cope with the wide scope of services available to them. We must tell those with the purse-strings that the problems will not go away, much as many would like them to do. In fact, with acute paediatric medical care being now so improved and sophisticated, many children are now surviving with a mental or physical disability who would previously have died. As doctors, we should be urging government and other institutions to better identify the magnitude of the problem. The days are long passed when the mentally disabled should be kept behind closed doors. That this still happens in Hong Kong cannot be doubted — even to the casual visitor the number of handicapped children seen on the streets is much less than in many other countries. Shame and guilt continue to haunt and destroy many families with mentally disabled members. Our responsibilities to improve public awareness is imperative. But before we do this, we need to put our own house in order to educate ourselves, and what better place to start than with a new generation of medical students who have for too long previously been constrained in their medical education to hospital-orientated problems of childhood. Spending time with these children in school, living and talking to them, will create the empathy which is so needed — an approach that in our department at the Prince of Wales Hospital we are trying to foster.

Conclusion

I end on a rather dismal note. What of these children when they lose their childhood appeal and enter the adult arena. After leaving special schools, following often many years of education, many withdraw again behind a cloak of obscurity in the home. Contact with these children is often lost so that any feedback is incomplete. What we do know is that far too many regress into apathy and helplessness. How about our ideals now? At the age of 16 there is an insufficient choice of post-school placement and vocational preparation for school-leavers to prepare them for open/sheltered employment. There are only limited numbers of places in Vocational Training Centres, Sheltered Workshops and Work Activity Centres for them. The problem is especially acute for moderate and severe grade students. In a survey in January 1985 of the schools belonging to the Hong Kong Association for the Mentally Handicapped, about 50% of school-leavers graduates were awaiting placement from home. What then medical duties and responsibilities to the adult mentally handicapped? What about their physical health? How hard are we pressing for improvements in further amenities for students when they leave school in sheltered workshops, training centres, work activity centres to provide further education, retraining opportunities, programmes on leisure, sex education and recreational

Figure 2. Mentally Handicapped Adults in a Sheltered Workshop: Too Few Opportunities?

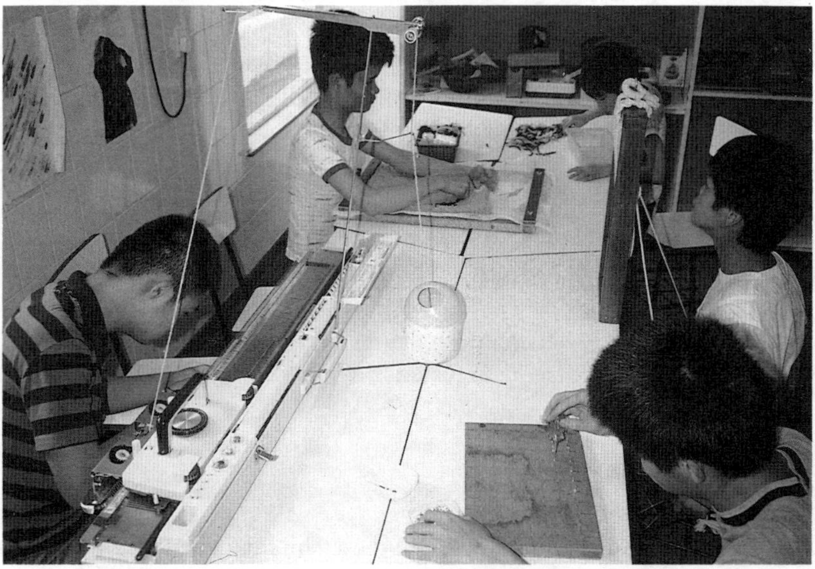

and social training? Without continued opportunities, the skills that have been learned will enter attrition. With modern medicine, death in childhood is now uncommon and numbers of mentally handicapped adults are increasing. Can we as a community manage? Have we the maturity of wisdom to accept the existence and the needs of these persons?

One of the greatest challenges facing our medical community at the present time is not in the ever-increasing complexity of applying modern technology to the diagnosis and treatment of illness. It is to continue to lift the veil of almost embarrassed silence from the heads of the disabled and provide them with a dignity and opportunity that regrettably even in the mid-1980s is still accorded to too few. We have the responsibility to tell the public that they need not fear the mentally handicapped; that they are people as you and I; that they have feelings and emotions though these may not be expressed as you and I might do so; that they have every right to recreation and protection and other facilities; that however disabled, they might have the right to dignity.

Acknowledgements

I wish to thank Miss Juliet Lee for her immense patience with me in the preparation and typing of this manuscript.

Further Reading

1. Special Educational Needs. Report of the Committee of Enquiry into the Education of Handicapped Children and Young People. Chairman, Mrs. H. M. Warnock. London: HMSO, 1978.
2. Zigler, E., Balla, D., and Hodapp, P. On the Definition and Classification of Mental Retardation. *Am J Ment Defic*, 1984; 89:215–30.
3. The Causes of Severe Mental Handicap (Annotation). *Dev Med Child Neurol*, 1982; 24:386–93.

Epilogue

Occidental and Oriental Variations: Reflections on Paediatric Morbidity in Hong Kong and Britain

Introduction

In 1982 when I first arrived in Hong Kong to work, I had presumed that in a part of the world where the ravages of poverty, malnutrition and infectious diseases belonged largely to the past, the clinical problems in children would be not that dissimilar from those in Britain, except for some obvious genetic disorders.

As a general statement I was to find this to be true but in quite a short time I also came to appreciate the existence of many intriguing and unexpected variations in morbidity, some subtle, others less so, which reflected genetic influences and, never to be underestimated, the impact of lifestyle and socio-economic conditions on the growing child. The fascinating variations that gradually unfolded came to have important educational repercussions beyond their biological interest since to be meaningful and relevant, undergraduate and postgraduate teaching needed to emphasize these variations. With few exceptions, most textbooks in Hong Kong are written by paediatricians practising in Western countries with often little regard for geographical variations in the pattern of illness.

Returned now to paediatric practice in Britain and tuned once more into the problems of children here, these variations in morbidity have become even more vivid to me. Some of these I have chosen to reflect on in this final chapter, but not in any way as an exhaustive compendium of all possible clinical disorders that might vary in their incidence between the Occident and the Orient. I have chosen those conditions with particularly striking variations or which hold a certain intrigue for me.

Genetic Disorders

It is common knowledge that the genetic disorder most frequently encountered in children in Hong Kong, in common with other countries in Southeast Asia, is *glucose–6–phosphate dehydrogenase (G–6–PD) deficiency*: 4.4% of males and 0.4% of females have been estimated to be affected.[1] Not so long ago, this disorder was a dreadful scourge that contributed significantly to death in the new-born period, and in the long term, to severe neuro-developmental disability from kernicterus. Many paediatricians practising in Hong Kong still have vivid memories of these times. In 1971, cord blood screening was introduced to a couple of hospitals and then in 1984, G–6–PD screening, using a quantitative assay of the enzyme activity on cord blood, was introduced throughout the territory under the direction of the Clinical Genetic Service of the then Medical and Health Department. Now, mothers and fathers of all diagnosed babies are advised how to prevent the occurrence of haemolytic crises in their children, guidance further reinforced during routine attendance's at maternal and child health (MCH) clinics. The effectiveness of this screening programme is, without a doubt, one of the major medical triumphs to have been achieved in Hong Kong in the last couple of decades: admission to paediatric wards of children with haemolytic crises being now very uncommon.

Thalassaemic syndromes are the most common autosomal recessive conditions. *α-thalassaemia* is still an important cause of stillbirth and each year approximately 25 infants are born with *β-thalassaemia major* requiring lifelong regular blood transfusions and subcutaneous iron chelation only to suffer and die in later adolescence and early adult life from serious irreversible multiple system disease. The *β-thalassaemia trait*, prevalence about 2.5%, accounts for many children having an incidental finding of haemoglobin below 11 g/dl, but rarely symptomatic and not requiring treatment.[2]

Of genetic disorders not seen in Hong Kong compared to Britain, *phenylketonuria* (PKU) and *cystic fibrosis* (CF) are those most conspicuously absent. The story of PKU is especially intriguing. A study in the early 1970s of about 18,000 new-born babies screened in the new-born period did not turn up any case of PKU (Dr. Henrietta Ip, unpublished data), seeming to confirm local paediatric claims that PKU is not found in Hong Kong. A contrary opinion, however, emanates from parts of mainland China, especially Shanghai, Beijing and Guangzhou, where PKU has apparently been diagnosed and leading to neonatal screening programmes being implemented. One such study from the First Affiliated Hospital of Beijing Medical University of 198,320 new-borns screened by Guthrie's bacterial inhibition assay found an overall incidence of 1/16,500, a rate similar to those found in Caucasian populations.[3] I did however meet some sceptism in Hong Kong over these findings where PKU is not included in the neonatal screening programme, new-born screening being confined to G–6–PD deficiency and congenital hypothyroidism (using cord blood TSH). (This latter condition incidentally has an incidence similar to that reported in Caucasian and other Asiatic populations of about 1 in 3,500.[4]) I did not come across any child in schools and institutions for the mentally handicapped whom I could recall with hair fairer than usual and anything other than dark brown eyes, claims that have been made in some parts of China. The history of China during the Mongolian Empire records a sizeable population of "coloured eye" people inhabiting principally North China. Distinguishable from the Han people from the Yellow River area, these people, mostly Persians and Indians, could conceivably have introduced the gene for PKU into the country. But enough of anthropological speculation!

It is intriguing how CF, the commonest serious autosomal recessive genetic disorder in Caucasian populations, seems also not to have been described in the Chinese. But it has been reported in Japan.[5] With the recent cloning and sequencing of the gene responsible for CF, the reason for the absence of this disease might soon be explained. Could it be that there is an abnormal mutation of the gene in the Chinese but not the one that results in the characteristic phenotype?

Conditions Determined before Birth

Preaxial polydactyly is much more common in Hong Kong.[6] The spectrum of congenital heart disease is also slightly different with *univentricular heart* and *severe right ventricular outflow obstruction* in the new-born more common and *left heart abnormalities — aortic stenosis, hypoplastic left heart, aortic coarctation* — less common than in Caucasian populations.[7,8] Remarkable in its virtual absence is *spina bifida* (anencephaly does occur but usually as part of syndromes of multiple congenital anomalies).

A study from Tsan Yuk Hospital of the incidence of neural tube defects among all deliveries in 1961–80 (123,491 births) showed incidences of anencephaly, spina bifida and encephalocoele 0.83, 0.12 and 0.06 per 1,000 births respectively,[9] rates noted at the time to be similar to those reported from Singapore, Thailand and Manila. Comparable incidences of spina bifida in the United Kingdom were then 1.5–4.1/1,000. Between 1984 and 1990 in the Prince of Wales Hospital,* and covering about 30,000 births, there were 15 cases of anencephaly, 2 of encephalocoele, 3 of meningomyelocele (all in South Asian babies), and 2 of meningocele (Dr. T. F. Fok, personal communication).

The Southern Chinese diet typically is rich in green vegetables, fresh fruit and rice, thereby providing a substantial amount of folic acid. Methods of cooking vegetables (rapid stir frying or by brief steaming) would be expected to preserve folic acid content better than Western cooking practices where vegetables are often overcooked in boiling water. Apparently in North China, spina bifida is as common as it used to be in many Western countries (Professor Michael Lawrence, personal communication). In these regions, diet is influenced by season and fresh vegetables are scarce for much of the year. Some Chinese medical opinion has linked this higher incidence of spina bifida with a much lower folic acid intake.[10] All this does more than provide a hint that the Southern Chinese could be protected by their diet from abnormal neural tube embryogenesis, supporting the currently held view that folic acid sufficiency is needed to prevent the expression of genetic predisposition to neural tube defects.

Later gestation gave the impression of providing further protection for the fetus. I found *intra-uterine growth retardation* to be much less common, the thin scraggy, "small-for-dates" baby being an unusual sight. The ratio of mid-arm circumference to occipital frontal circumference, an index of late gestation growth retardation, is significantly higher than in Asian, white and black neonates in London.[11] There is also a lower incidence of *very low birth-weight* in Hong Kong, Lau and his colleagues in 1984

---

* Many observations in this chapter derive from paediatric experiences in the Prince of Wales Hospital (PWH) from the time of its opening in 1984 to when I left in 1989. Over these years, we established a method of clinical audit that provided a useful objective account of our clinical experiences (see Reference 35).

describing an incidence of infants weighing < 1,500 g at birth of 6.9/1,000,[12] considerably lower than the 14.4/1,000 described over the same period in England and Wales. But such low incidences are not peculiar to Hong Kong Chinese, being reported also in Shanghai[13] and in Chinese populations in Australia.[14]

I suggest these more favourable intra-uterine conditions are related to social factors and less maternal hypertensive disease. Teenage pregnancies are still uncommon in Hong Kong; smoking and alcohol consumption during pregnancy very unusual; diet in pregnancy excellent and antenatal care in the MCH clinics and hospital very strictly supervised and full advantage taken by most pregnant mothers. Hypertension in pregnancy is also less common in the Chinese.[14] A fascinating study in 1987 by Dr. Andrew Lyon from the British Military Hospital showed a significantly increased risk of pregnancy hypertension in mothers from Britain compared to Hong Kong.[15] Lyon emphasized the great care that had to be taken in drawing too many conclusions from his study because of the Chinese and British groups being not strictly comparable, but nonetheless his findings do provide some interesting pointers. Others have also drawn attention to an under-representation in Chinese mothers of risk factors commonly associated with preterm delivery and growth retardation.[13,14] Hence, I speculate, a safer intra-uterine environment for the baby.

Indeed, I vividly recall the words of paediatrician I met in Guangzhou in 1985 when visiting one of the medical schools in that city who had then only recently returned from a couple of years neonatal attachment in a busy North American city. Discussing some of the problems of neonatal care, especially the virtual absence of very small babies in her unit, her response was that China had yet to witness those particular social and environmental problems that contribute so much to neonatal morbidity in the West. As a general statement, I considered the same to also apply in Hong Kong where, compared with many parts of the developed world, the social soil seems less fertile for the seeds of extreme prematurity and growth retardation to germinate. What is not appreciated is that since the early 1960s when mortality data began officially to be gathered, perinatal and neonatal mortalities in Hong Kong have been consistently lower than in Britain. In 1965, a time when environmental conditions in Hong Kong were extremely harsh for so many of its people, perinatal mortality was 23/1,000 compared with about 31/1,000 in Britain;[16] this provides further support for my contention that some inherent protection is conferred upon the Chinese baby before birth. It would also be expected to follow that long-term neuro-developmental handicap would be less common but as yet population statistics are unavailable to record the incidence of cerebral palsy and other perinatally determined neuro-developmental handicap.

Problems in the New-born

All babies in Hong Kong, born either in hospital or in one of 47 MCH clinics scattered throughout the territory, have a thorough neonatal examination. Out of this emerges the intriguing finding of a very low incidence of *congenital dislocation of the hip*, at least ten times less common than in Caucasians.[17] One explanation from recent ultrasound studies is that acetabular morphology of the hip joint in Chinese babies is more favourable, causing less potential instability.[18]

But without doubt, and paediatricians in Hong Kong need no reminding of this, the most common clinical problem in the new-born is *neonatal jaundice* which, in its non-haemolytic type, is especially prevalent in Chinese babies. 50–78% of normal term infants in Hong Kong have a serum bilirubin level > 171 mmol/L (10 mg/dl).[19] Reasons for such a high incidence of jaundice, that I used to consider of the "exaggerated" physiological type, an imbalance between production and excretion of bilirubin, is unknown. In 1984, a study from Singapore where jaundice among Chinese babies is also very common showed a significant association between elevated cord blood alpha-feto protein and subsequent jaundice in full-term normal babies, inferring an immaturity of hepatic enzyme conjugating mechanisms.[20] A study in Hong Kong in 1984 suggested that a slightly increased rate of haemolysis, as measured by carbon monoxide excretion, could be contributory.[21] Another view has been that jaundice could be associated with mothers consuming certain herbal medicines during pregnancy, a tradition still popular in Hong Kong where many of these herbs are held to have beneficial effects on the process of childbirth.[22] In times past, new-born babies were also often given herbs by their mothers to help rid them of "placental toxins," a practice, though much less common, that still prevails, especially in the older parts of Hong Kong. *In vitro* studies by Professor C. Y. Yeung and his colleagues at Queen Mary Hospital have shown that a very popular herb, *Cheun-Lin*, can displace bilirubin from its albumen-binding sites,[19] but which of the thirty or so ingredients is the active principle is not known. In a 1985 study from Tsan Yuk Hospital, 54% of about 10,600 mothers admitted to multiple herb consumption during pregnancy.[22] But contrary to other reports, and further complicating the issue, there was no significant association between maternal herb consumption during pregnancy and the extent of neonatal hyperbilirubinaemia: neither were G–6–PD deficient babies more severely jaundiced as a consequence of herb consumption by the mother. The intriguing association between herbs and neonatal jaundice has yet to be resolved and I have little doubt this will be the subject of much continued research.

The continuing very high incidence of neonatal jaundice led to the transcutaneous bilirubinometer being introduced in several of the major hospitals throughout Hong Kong in the early 1980s and also in MCH clinics as a reliable and non-invasive means of assessing jaundice.[23] But fortunately no longer is jaundice the devastating scourge it used to be. It is worthwhile being reminded for example that in 1971 in the University Paediatric Unit, Queen Mary Hospital, 8.7% of term infants with neonatal jaundice developed kernicterus.[19] Phototherapy, introduced about twenty years ago, has radically changed the face of jaundice: exchange transfusions are now rarely needed. In PWH of about 100 term jaundiced infants treated each month with phototherapy, exchange transfusion was needed on average on only one or two occasions (Dr. T. F. Fok, personal communication). It is held also that somehow socio-economic improvement has contributed significantly to this dramatic decline in severe jaundice (Professor C. Y. Yeung, personal communication). Neonatal jaundice persists not so much a worrying medical problem but one more of social irritation causing separation of baby from mother in the early weeks following delivery with all its inconveniences, high bed occupancy in the neonatal nurseries and a huge primary care burden for doctors and nurses working in the territory's many MCH clinics.[24]

I cannot leave the new-born period without mentioning the tremendous achievement in the 1980s of the interruption of perinatal transmission of the hepatitis-B virus (HBV) at birth by early vaccination and passive immunization. There is an appalling toll in Southeast Asia from the HBV carrier state with hepatocellular carcinoma, hepatic cirrhosis, carcinoma of the stomach, the causes of so much premature death in middle life. Many countries in Asia have now confirmed the perinatal period as the most important time for transmitting HBV, resulting in carrier status. In Hong

Kong, all pregnant women are checked for HBV antigen status during antenatal visits. Babies of carrier mothers are given HBIg together with a first dose of vaccine at birth followed by two further doses of vaccine at 1 and 4 months (a routine now given to all babies of non-carrier mothers). Almost at a stroke, the devastation caused by the carrier state one generation from now will have been virtually eliminated.

Problems in Infancy and Childhood

As a prelude to mentioning some of the variations in morbidity of infants and older children, I would like to pause briefly on some aspects of their nutritional state, this being an important determinant of health in the young growing child.

With childhood mortality rates in the 1980s ranked alongside the best in Western countries, it was a surprise for me to discover when first I arrived that substantial local opinion held that undernutrition, especially of energy, calcium, vitamin D and iron intakes, was a continuing problem.[25] My immediate impression was that children looked a little smaller than those in Britain but they did not give the impression of being undernourished. A five-year longitudinal study in our department of growth and nutrition in babies born in the urban area of Sha Tin showed that between 6 and 18 months, there were certainly downward deviations in weight gain, and height and head circumference growth viewed against the National Centre of Health Statistics (NCHS) reference curves,[26,27] and skinfold thickness growth also showed much less adiposity than in Caucasian infants.[28] Yet intakes of major nutrients were all well within recommended dietary recommendations.[26,29,30] One fascinating feeding practice commented on very little was the regular use by mothers of compound herb preparations when reconstituting milk formula,[31] a practice believed to stimulate the baby's appetite, enhance absorption of nutrients from the gastrointestinal tract and help eliminate excess endogenous heat.

These very distinctive growth profiles in well-nourished children, and which are also found in children in many other healthy Asiatic populations,[32] led us to question the advisability of using the NCHS curves as a suitable reference for Southern Chinese children. We were concerned that reluctance to recognize adequate nutritional status could lead all too easily to overfeeding and a shift-away from the excellent Cantonese diet, nutritionally so well-balanced with its low intake of saturated fats (30% of the total energy content[33] compared with approximately 50% in the diet of British children[34] and refined carbohydrates and high fibre and protein). But I still have one nagging worry. Can I say that Hong Kong infants are well-nourished when so few are breast-fed? Of about 25% put to breast at birth in our study (a fairly typical sample of Hong Kong infants), only 8%, 6% and 2% were still breast-feeding at 2, 4 and 6 months respectively.[27] Very low rates of breast-feeding are widespread throughout Hong Kong (due chiefly to misconceptions held by mothers over the value of breast-feeding; ready availability of approved milk formula; the need and desire to return to work soon after delivery; short maternity leave; lack of privacy and an urgent lifestyle) and also in other newly industrialized countries of Southeast Asia. The economically rich Orient is neglecting breast-feeding. Is there a future cost?

Gastrointestinal Disease

Gastroenteritis, due chiefly to rotavirus, accounted for about 14% of all paediatric admissions to PWH in the mid-1980s.[35] But, as now in Britain and many other Western countries, most of these children were admitted for medically trivial reasons: gastroenteritis is no longer a serious medical problem. Rarely were babies seriously dehydrated on admission to hospital. Because of a higher incidence of genetically determined deficiency of lactase in Chinese, *secondary lactose intolerance* might be expected to frequently complicate gastroenteritis: surprisingly it was rare, no more common than in Britain. Far more frequent were iatrogenic complications of the treatment of gastroenteritis by outside practitioners, paralytic ileus and electrolyte disturbances from treatment with anti-motility drugs being not infrequent in children admitted to hospital. These therapeutic practices are now virtually extinct, thankfully, in Britain.

It was intriguing how uncommon *pyloric stenosis* was. During the 1970s and 1980s, the incidence in Britain was approximately 5/1,000.[36] In 1986–91, there were only 14 cases seen at PWH (approximately 0.27/1,000. Dr. K. Liu, personal communication). *Coeliac disease* does not occur in the Southern Chinese (although I have been told of some evidence from North China, where wheat is consumed more than in the predominantly rice-consuming south, that this disorder is known there). *Failure to thrive* was not a common hospital problem: adverse social factors at home and poor parenting skills were not the associated risk factors they are so often found to be here, an example of the protection afforded to the young infant by support within the family that is still a strong feature of Hong Kong life in spite of its high degree of urbanization. In older children, the chronic bowel inflammatory diseases, *ulcerative colitis* and *Crohn's disease*, are non-existent, as indeed are they in adults. Hong Kong is far from a Garden of Eden for the paediatric gastroenterologist!

Cot Death

I was very surprised when I first went to Hong Kong to discover how little aware were paediatricians there about the *sudden infant death syndrome* (SIDS — cot death). I first drew attention to this in a retrospective study published in the *Lancet* in 1985.[37] But Hong Kong was not alone in having such little awareness of SIDS. Paediatricians in China and other Southeast Asian countries confirmed a similar very low incidence. (In America, the incidence of SIDS had also been reported as lowest in the Asians.[38]) In a prospective study between 1 December 1986 and 31 November 1987 covering 70,519 births, only 21 cases of cot death were recorded in the whole of Hong Kong, an incidence of 0.29/1,000.[39] Comparable incidences in Britain were then about 2–4/1,000. To explain this much lower incidence, we wondered whether the "microenvironment" of Hong Kong infants, crowded living conditions leading to babies never being left alone (a marked contrast to the solitary sleeping habits of so many Western babies) might somehow protect, perhaps though an influence on respiratory control at a particularly vulnerable developmental stage. We wondered also, as have others since,[40,41] whether supine sleeping might also protect: traditionally Chinese babies in Hong Kong are seldom put to lie in the prone position for fear of suffocation. 44% of the index babies in our study compared with 7% of controls had this sleeping posture.[39] What I did learn in Hong Kong is that supine lying does not increase risks of aspiration of vomit, as has until recently been taught in Britain. Ethnic variations in the incidence of SIDS have also recently been shown in Britain. For example its incidence among Bangladeshi people, who for many other disorders in childhood are a high-risk population, is much lower than for the ethnic majority.[42]

These observations do more than hint that protective influences possibly exist for cot death that are linked with cultural attitudes to infant care. Might child care practices be playing a more decisive role than previously thought in aetiology of what is in Western countries still the commonest cause of post-neonatal death? A comment in the *Lancet* of 1987 by the Belgian Dr. Odent after visiting China in 1977 where the concept of cot death was virtually unknown among professional is worthwhile recalling. "Cot death is a disease of babies who spent their nights in an atmosphere of loneliness and that cot death is a disease of societies where the nuclear family has taken over."[43] I believe there is somewhere an "ethnic-geographical" clue to help us understand better the aetiology of SIDS and it is now well overdue that we look at cot death in a more anthropological perspective.

Iron and Vitamin D Deficiencies

Iron deficiency still arouses concern in Britain with reported prevalences of 12–45% in major urban areas[44] and especially common in non-white children. Held responsible are poor weaning diets and widespread consumption of pasteurized cows milk with its negligible amount of iron and risks of causing gastrointestinal blood loss.[45] In Hong Kong, and in spite of concern in the recent past about dietary deficiencies of iron, calcium and vitamin D during weaning, we were able to show virtually no iron deficiency (< 2%) at 18 months when weaning had been largely completed.[29] There was also no nutritional *vitamin D deficiency*[31] other than in some Vietnamese children and those more recently arrived from mainland China. With MCH clinics recommending affordable iron and vitamin fortified formulae as breast-milk substitutes well into the second year along with an excellent weaning diet and exposure to plenty of sunshine, it is not surprising that what are still among the most common nutritional deficiencies in so many other parts of the world, developed and developing alike, are so infrequent in Hong Kong.

Miscellaneous Conditions

Kawasaki disease is far more common than in Britain[46] although with nowhere near the high incidence of Japan. As an example 55 children were diagnosed in PWH between 1987 and 1990 (Dr. D. Leung, personal communication). I was surprised to find *myasthenia gravis* in young children occurring more frequently than in Caucasians. With its early onset, mild nature, frequent spontaneous remission rates and good prognosis[47] it is limited mostly to fatiguability of the ocular muscles. Children usually present with ptosis and ophthalmoplegia and sometimes as young as two years of age. There is a strong association with the histocompatibility complex HLA-DRW9, a genetically determined variant occurring more often in Chinese.[48]

Children presenting with extrapyramidal dyskinetic symptoms, *oculogyric crises*, caused by drugs often prescribed by general practitioners such as stemetil (prescribed for upper respiratory symptom) and metoclopramide (for vomiting) and complications of some Chinese medicinal treatments were commonly seen.[49] Their prompt recognition in Accident and Emergency Departments as a cause of bizarre acute neurological symptoms was important since intravenous diphenhydramine would rapidly reverse the symptoms and avoid unnecessary investigations and undesirable admission to hospital. Indeed, drug-induced extrapyramidal syndromes had always to be suspected in the differential diagnosis of any usual acute neurological problem in young children. In some instances, these were complications of a particular Chinese herb treatment, Bo Ying Pills,[49] the widely used Chinese medicine made up of nine active ingredients, recommended for cramps, high fever, coughs, insomnia and many other non-specific symptoms. Some of these ingredients could have caused extrapyramidal effects, but there was also the possibility that certain drugs were added to this medicine and responsible for the symptoms.

Acute post-streptococcal glomerulonephritis is still far more common than in Britain, though *rheumatic fever*, the other important streptococcal-related illness, is exceedingly rare. (Over five years [1984–89], only two children were diagnosed in PWH to have rheumatic fever in contrast to 216 with acute nephritis.) Of 74 children with acute nephritis admitted over an 18-month period in 1984–86 preceding streptococcal infection was as much in the skin as in the throat.[50] Barely a month would go by without a child being admitted with serious *upper gastrointestinal bleeding*; one study from the Division of Paediatric Surgery, Queen Mary Hospital, recorded as many as 49 children admitted with upper gastrointestinal haemorrhage between 1985 and 1988.[51] This bleeding in young children was usually attributed to multiple superficial gastric erosions and there was more than a high index of suspicion to blame aspirin and steroids contained in some medications prescribed outside hospital. *Systemic lupus erythematosus* (SLE) is well recognized to occur more often in Chinese people[52] and this was evident in Hong Kong hospital paediatric practice, girls particularly being affected. A serious multiple system disease SLE is a common cause of end stage renal failure in Hong Kong. In contrast, *insulin dependent diabetes mellitus* was much less common.

I am still coming to terms with the great concern in Britain about *child abuse* and the enormous range of problems encapsulated by this diagnosis. The first case of child abuse in Hong Kong was officially documented in 1979 and since then its manifold physical and emotional components have increasingly become a major focus of medical and social concern. There is no systematic documentation of its incidence but there is no doubt that non-accidental physical injury — bruises, burns, bites, lacerations, fractures, subdural haematoma etc., problems that have been increasingly recognized in Britain over the past 30 years is very much less common. In PWH, only 38 children were admitted in the three-year period 1984–87 suffering confirmed or strongly suspected non-accidental injury[53] and I have no reason to believe that this was then anything other than an accurate reflection of the situation throughout Hong Kong. Most of the abuse was physical, and related especially to disciplining older children (in our study only eight were under five years old), and exacted chiefly for disobedience or misconduct at home. There was only one possible instance of sexual abuse. Underachievement would sometimes be the flashpoint for child-beating, but this was sometimes viewed as acceptable practice. Many children in whom physical abuse was diagnosed had been born in Hong Kong, sent to China to be brought up by relatives only to return unknown to the parents who in turn failed to cope with stresses posed by a young child rejoining the family.

An appropriate comparison to this experience in Britain is in a 1990 paper from Leeds, population of about 750,000 (fewer than the one million or so population then served by PWH), where between 1985 and 1988, 769 children with physical abuse and 949 with sexual abuse were diagnosed.[54] I am not naive enough to deny the possibility that the real incidence of child abuse in Hong Kong could be more than it gave the impression of being (especially perhaps in the massive housing estates in the New Territories where many young families are now being housed, many miles away from their families in the older urban areas of Hong Kong and Kowloon). But even allowing this possibility, it was nowhere near the magnitude it is now in Britain. But why? A very large number of families live in extremely overcrowded living conditions that would not be tolerated in Britain, even in the most disadvantaged council estate. Paradoxically perhaps might "opportunities" for abuse be less. The extended family is still very strong in Hong Kong with tremendous support given by other family members to mothers and young children who are highly cherished and valued: this could be preventing abuse. There are virtually no unmarried mothers, few teenage pregnancies and almost full employment, factors that could also provide an umbrella of protection.

Enuresis and *encopresis*, in Britain, often considered social and behavioural problems, were seen much less often in out-patient and MCH clinics. A community study in 1987 in Sha Tin of 2,500 children aged 3–7 attending normal kindergartens and primary schools revealed that 84%, 98% and virtually 100% of the children were reported by their parents to be dry at 3, 6 and 7 years respectively.[55] This compared then with prevalence from multiple data on children from Britain, Western Europe, Australia and North America between 1956 and 1969 of 68%, 84% and 89% of children at similar ages being dry at night.[56] At the same time, it was also my impression that in Hong Kong parents were much less concerned about bedwetting even when it did occur. I am still curious why bedwetting is such an uncommon problem there: adverse environmental factors, including unsatisfactory housing, have been quoted an *unfavourable* variable in militating against successful treatment of bedwetting.[57]

Infectious diseases occurred sporadically, affected children usually being referred to the Infectious Disease Unit in Princess Margaret Hospital in Kowloon. The most common communicable diseases were viral hepatitis and bacillary dysentery, resulting usually from food contamination. With impressive immunization uptakes, rates varying from 88 to 99% in 1988–89,[58] outbreaks of measles and whooping cough were exceedingly rare. I cannot also recall seeing or hearing about any child with a serious complication of pertussis immunization. *Human immunodeficiency virus* (HIV) infection was confined to the haemophiliac population. In 1987, 40% of haemophiliac children possessed the HIV antibody (Dr. N. K. Leung, personal communication). Perinatally acquired HIV infection had yet to be described in Hong Kong when I was there.

One very interesting feature given the high population density of urban living in Hong Kong was the virtual absence of *meningococcal meningitis*. H. Influenzae was the commonest cause of bacterial meningitis. Of 61 patients aged 4 days to 11 years with bacterial meningitis admitted to one of the paediatric units at Princess Margaret Hospital between 1979 and 1985, there was not one case of meningococcal meningitis (Dr. N. K. Leung, personal communication). Our experience in PWH mirrored this, not one case of meningococcal meningitis being diagnosed in 1984–89. Between 1986 and 1988, there were only 14 notified cases of "cerebrospinal meningitis" and meningococcal infection in the whole of Hong Kong, adults and children combined.[59] Reasons for the extremely low incidence of meningococcal disease are not known. Might it be that crowded living conditions from birth produce from a very early age a protective antibody response in the whole population?

I would like finally to turn to some disorders that impressed me as having an incidence that showed no obvious differences between West and East. *Acute respiratory tract infections*, of upper and lower respiratory passages, were very common reasons for hospital admission. Audit of admissions to the paediatric wards of the PWH in 1984–88 showed lower respiratory tract infections accounting for 41% of admissions.[35] In recent years, and in common with many other countries, there has been reported in Hong Kong an increased prevalence of *asthma* with many more children requiring hospital admission.[60] *Febrile convulsions* were as common. *Urinary tract infections* were also much the same and presented in the usual way. *Normal variant short stature* was as much a problem but without the "indulgence" of being able to treat these children with growth hormone. *Neuromuscular disorders* and *neuro-developmental handicap* gave an impression of being no less common than in Britain, but exact statistics are not available. As paediatrician to a school of nearly 300 severely mentally handicapped children where I used to conduct weekly "primary care" clinics and responsible also for continued care of the children, I did not discern any obvious difference in the spectrum of the major causes of handicap. But some of the most distressing children were orphans who at some stage had been labelled as mentally handicapped, not for any obvious physical reason but as a consequence of abandonment, lack of care and stimulation and behavioural disturbance acquired through their own emotional conflicts during passages between orphanages and other centres and institutions. Disturbed they might be, underachieving their potential they undoubtedly were, but mentally handicapped they were not. For as long as this label remained around their necks, the solution to their problem through adoption was difficult. Over the years, I became more encouraged to find fewer of these so labelled and some normal kindergartens had begun to accept these children.

In recent years, the problems of the *chronic multiple handicapped child* have become increasingly a concern in Hong Kong. For too long tucked away out of sight, these children are now being recognized for what they are and for what they need. But I felt there was still too little awareness of the multiple physical, educational, behavioural and social problems of these children. Hopefully the much greater exposure now being given to the current generation of medical students will reap rewards in future years to improve the outlook for these children.

Conclusion

In February 1990, a leading article in the *Lancet* expressed many anxieties over the troubled state of the hospital services in Hong Kong.[61] At the same time as sharing and understanding much of this worry, I did express in a letter to that same journal a concern that amid all the gloom and doom not one word of credit was given to major achievements in health care in Hong Kong accomplished in the face of what must be seen to many as almost impossible odds.[62]

The people of Hong Kong are the last who need to be told of the immense changes that have taken place in the past thirty years or so in its social and economic environment as it has emerged as one of Asia's most rapidly developing newly industrialized regions, expanding its population from 0.5 million in 1945 to six million in 1990. One highly significant marker of these changes are improvements in childhood mortality that have taken place. In 1956, infant mortality was 60.9/1,000; in 1989 it was 6.9/1,000.[58] Perinatal and neonatal mortalities in 1989 were 7.6/1,000 and 4.8/1,000 respectively and under five mortality 8.2/1,000. What is especially remarkable is that these impressive improvements have taken place in the face of periodic influxes of huge numbers of people from mainland China caused by various social upheavals in that country, migrations that I have no doubt would have dealt a crippling blow to the health and social services of most nations.

The sorry plight of children in Hong Kong as little as a generation ago was vividly described by Professor Elaine Field and Dr. Flora Baber in their classic monograph *Growing Up in Hong Kong*[63] (What a pity this book is not more widely read in Hong Kong. It was, as an epidemiological study, way before its time). Described in the book were the appalling living conditions of thousands of children in the 1960s, their meagre nutritional state and their affliction by widespread scourges of infections and infectious diseases. But how times have changed. Living conditions, through remarkable economic achievements, have improved beyond recognition. An outstanding Maternal and Child Heath Service has (though still too often under-appreciated) contributed much to improve the physical well-being of mothers during pregnancy, the safety of childbirth, and the health of children by immunization, physical and developmental surveillance, nutrition advice and general primary health care. The increased secular trend in physical size of Hong Kong children over the past twenty or so years of record-keeping is further testimony to these improvements.[64,65] Hospital facilities for sick children, including services for the new-born, have also improved immeasurably (although not perhaps as rapidly as many would wish) and there has emerged a very high overall standard of paediatric care both inside and outside hospital contributed also in no mean way by major expansions in postgraduate education and professional training programmes in which the University of Hong Kong, The Chinese University of Hong Kong, the government hospitals and the Hong Kong Paediatric Society have all played leading roles.

My professional and personal involvement with paediatrics in all sectors of the Health Service during my years in Hong Kong have made me respect deeply what has been achieved in the field of Child Health, even more so now that I can view these achievements from a distance. I am sure that there are similar accomplishments in other medical and health fields. In a historical context to provide specialist hospital services before coping with basic social and public health needs has been a mistake committed in all too many developing countries. In Hong Kong, with its population density and unique set of problems, I believe it was wholly appropriate for initial priorities to have been given to improve public health and primary care. That cost a lot of money, which may be an important reason for the exhausted state of much of the hospital services in Hong Kong, a point not conceded by harsh critics of its Medical Services.

But, and I say this with some trepidation, perhaps success had come too quickly for comfort. The major achievements in the health and welfare of children have been made virtually within one generation: in most parts of the Western world such progress took several generations. Expectations of doctors, other health workers and the public, fuelled by a high level of education attainment in the population, are overextending the abilities of the health services to provide specialized hospital care. Frustrations are further exacerbated by the expectations of those who have undergone postgraduate training outside Hong Kong. But I must put on record that many of these problems in Hong Kong are also shared in hospitals in the more traditionally wealthy countries. I returned to work in Britain at a time of the most vigorous reforms in the National Health Service that have been instituted since its beginnings in 1947. Because of financial stringencies, we are now having to recognize far more so than ever before that provision of health care is not a bottomless pit which can, given the opportunity, consume the total gross national product. Priorities in health care are having to be made, many unpalatable. There are bed closures to better rationalize services. The length of out-patients lists in many parts of the country are a major concern. Junior medical staff are uncompromisingly demanding official recognition of a working week of no more than 72 hours by 1995. Market forces are being introduced into the health services with the evolution of provider/purchaser roles. Audit of clinical quality performance is now compulsory. Much greater emphasis is being given to public health and preventive medicine. I emphasize these developments to put some of the current worries in Hong Kong at least into some perspective, to make health professionals there realize that the world over there are concerns over future developments in hospital services.

But at the same time, I also recognize that many worries in Hong Kong are unique to its geo-political predicament, most notable being the "China Question" that is understandably all pervasive in directing future thinking of how the health services should develop and which suffered such devastating shake-up in the aftermath of the June 1989 Tiananmen Square disaster. It is all so easy to pass sweeping judgements from the smug safety of possessing a passport that allows one almost to be a voyeur of the scene of so much anxiety, fear and frustration felt by so many in Hong Kong. Hong Kong has very committed and able doctors, nurses and administrators and those in professions allied to medicine. Medical students are as well-educated as any, and hard working. It is therefore sad to realize that (though for very understandable reasons) for reasons of future personal security, many are seeking permanent dwelling beyond its shores. Hopefully many will return to Hong Kong once their future is found to be more secure. I am also told that fewer young people are now wishing to enter the medical and allied professions. Hong Kong must continue to recruit and keep its young people of vision, enthusiasm and public spirit, and who want to make things work in after all what is their home. Close links with academic and health institutes overseas must be maintained and built on. The new Hospital Authority and the Hong Kong Academy of Medicine will, I am sure, work together to see the emergence of an invigorated hospital service with better hospital provisions for patients, shorter out-patient lists, more civilized living and working conditions for medical and nursing staff, more satisfying training programmes, etc. Much has to be achieved (although these tasks must at times seem unsurmountable) yet I hope not at the expense of further improvements in services outside hospital, especially those for the elderly, disabled and terminally ill, and primary care in general. In child health I would like to think that this would in time be embraced by what we are trying to achieve in Britain through a combined child care service with hospital and community services working together in a "seamless" manner to give the best possible care to all children whatever their problems.

But amid all this shifting sand, there is one thing that Hong Kong must not fail to do. At this most critical time in its history, it must not fail to proclaim its many outstanding achievements that are all the more remarkable when viewed from the perspective of other countries in the region. I am proud to be able to have shared in some of these.

Addendum

This is a letter to the *Lancet* in response to an editorial in 1994 on the medical future for Hong Kong. (Reprinted by permission of the publisher: Davies, D. P. Medical Future for Hong Kong. *Lancet*, 1994; 344:1,641. © by The Lancet 1994.)

Medical Future for Hong Kong

"In your timely and thoughtful 29 October editorial on the future facing Hong Kong medicine, you assume that the only source of local medical graduates is the medical faculty of the University of Hong Kong. Another graduate source, The Chinese University of Hong Kong has since 1985 also produced doctors with a degree as well-recognized as that of the University of Hong Kong.

"Hong Kong is fortunate in being able to produce high-calibre graduates from its two medical schools. These graduates should provide the momentum to carry medicine in Hong Kong beyond 1997 into a new era, one more international than before — with its increasing close links with medical fraternities in Southeast Asia, China, Australia, New Zealand, North America, and Canada — as well as retaining important contact with British medical institutions. Even with the inevitable change in previous close links with the U.K. that will accompany political change in the colony in 1997, to deny that Britain and British doctors will still have a very special role and responsibility is to deny the closeness that has existed in the development of undergraduate and postgraduate medicine between the two communities for so many years. For those in this country who have a special feeling for Hong Kong, having respect for its medical profession and its medical practice and social commitment, we must make it known to our colleagues there that we are also available to help and support the evaluation of a new system of medicine.

"If the speed with which the Hong Kong Academy of Medicine was established a few years ago (and, beneath its umbrella its new specialist colleges,) is anything to go by the future is full of promise. But as is so often the case the major threat of Hong Kong will come from within. It is not sufficient for Hong Kong to train its own doctors, nurses, and other professionals in health-related fields. They must be retained. Continuing haemorrhage of its medical fraternity to other parts of the world will seriously threaten the development of medical care. Without appropriately trained people, high ideals become an empty shell. This surely is the main challenge, and the most difficult to overcome, to Hong Kong medicine that you do not sufficiently emphasize?"

Acknowledgements

I thank my many friends and professional colleagues in Hong Kong who over the years helped me gain a balanced perspective of the clinical problems of Chinese culminating in these final impressions. If any misperceptions and inaccuracies have crept into the text, I am solely to blame. For these I apologize.

References

1. Chau, A. S., Lam, Y. M., Lui, S., *et al.* Genetic Services in Hong Kong. *J Med Genet*, 1990; 27:380–83.

2. Lam, T. K., So, L. Y., Poon, S. H., *et al.* Prevalence of β-thalassaemia Trait in Hong Kong Children. *HK J Paediatr*, 1989; 6:119–21.
3. Liu Shen-ru, and Zuo Qi-jau. Newborn Screening for Phenylketonuria in Eleven Districts. *Chinese Med J*, 1986; 99:113–18.
4. Chan, V.S.M., and Lam, S.T.S. The Hong Kong Government Neonatal Screening Programme for Congenital Hypothyroidism (Abstract). *Proceedings of International Conference on Mental Retardation*. Hong Kong: The Hong Kong Medical and Health Department, April 1991.
5. Yamashiro, Y., Oguchi, S., Shimizu, T., *et al.* Neonatal Mass Screening of CF in Japan — A Preliminary Report. *Proceedings of International Conference on Cystic Fibrosis*. Melbourne, 1988. Abstract, G(b) 4; 21.
6. Chen, J.C.Y., Chow, S. K., and Leung, P. C. Classification of 578 Cases of Congenital Upper Limb Anomalies with the IFSSH System: A 10 Years Experience. *J Hand Surg*, 1987; 12:1,055–60.
7. Lo, N. S., Leung, P., and Lau, K. C. Pattern of Congenital Heart Disease in Hong Kong. *HK J Paediatr*, 1985; 2:188–93.
8. Sung, R.Y.T., So, L. Y., Ng, H. K., *et al.* Echocardiography as a Tool for Determining the Incidence of Congenital Heart Disease in Newborn Babies: A Pilot Study in Hong Kong. *Int J Cardiol*, 1991; 30:43–47.
9. Ghosh, A., Woo, J.S.K., Poon, I.M.L., *et al.* Neural Tube Defects in Hong Kong Chinese. *Lancet*, 1981; 2:244–45.
10. Ye, H. The Strategy of Risk Approach in Perinatal Care in Shuniyi County, Beijing. *Symposium on Paediatrics in China and Africa*. London: Royal Society of Medicine, June 1986.
11. Davies, D. P., Lui, S., Lo, L., *et al.* The Ratio of Mid-arm Circumference to Occipital Frontal Circumference in Chinese Babies: A Marker of Late Gestation Growth Retardation. *Early Hum Dev*, 1987; 15:329 32.
12. Lau, S. P., Au-Yeung, C. L., Yeung, B.W.Y., *et al.* Major Determinants of Neonatal Mortality in Hong Kong. *HK J Paediatr*, 1984; 1:22–29.
13. Chalmers, I. Shanghai. *Lancet*, 1980; 1:137–39.
14. Beischer, N. A., and Liang, S. T. A Glimpse at Chinese Obstetrics 1984 — Why Do Chinese Have a Low Incidence of Prematurity? *Aust NZ J Obstet Gynaec*, 1984; 24:233–34.
15. Lyon, A. J. Trends in Perinatal Mortality of British and Chinese Infants Delivered in the British Military Hospital, Hong Kong: 1976–85. *HK J Paediatr*, 1987; 4:20–27.
16. Lau, S. P., Davies, D. P., Fung, K. P., *et al.* Perinatal and Neonatal Morbidity in Hong Kong: An Appraisal. *J HK Med Assoc*, 1985; 37:1,342–44.
17. Hoaglund, F. T., Kalamchi, A., Poon, R., *et al.* Congenital Hip Dislocation and Dysplasia in Southern Chinese. *Int Orthop*, 1981; 4:243–46.
18. Chan, Y. L., Chen, J.C.Y., and Metreweli, C. Sonographic Evaluation of

Acetabular Morphometry in Chinese Infants — An Answer to the Relatively Low Incidence of Congenital Hip Dislocation in the Chinese. Abstract: 39 (p. 388), 27th Congress of the European Society of Paediatric Radiology, 1990.

19. Yeung, C. Y., Lee, F. T., and Wong, H. N. Effect of a Popular Chinese Herb on Neonatal Bilirubin Protein Binding. *Biol Neonate*, 1990; 58:98–103.
20. Tan, K. L., Loganath, A., Roy, A. C., *et al.* Cord Plasma α-Fetoprotein Values and Neonatal Jaundice. *Pediatrics*, 1984; 74:1,065–68.
21. Lau, S. P., Wong, K. H., Fung, K. P., *et al.* Carbon Monoxide Production and Neonatal Hyperbilirubinaemia. *HK J Paediatr*, 1985; 2:93–94.
22. Fok, T. F., Lau, S. P., and Hui, C. W. Chinese Herbs in Pregnancy and Neonatal Jaundice. *HK J Paediatr*, 1985; 2:138–44.
23. Sung, R.Y.T., Davies, D. P., and Simon, M.P.T. Transcutaneous Bilirubinometry: A Valuable Screening Method for Neonatal Jaundice. *HK J Paediatr*, 1985; 2:14–15.
24. Leung, S. L., Lai, P.Y.F., and Davies, D. P. A Survey of Work Undertaken in 1 Year by a Medical Officer Working in a Maternal and Child Health Clinic in Hong Kong: Implications for Training. *Ann Trop Paediatr*, 1990; 10:99–108.
25. Li, A.M.C., Baber, F. M., and Yu, A.M.C. Infant Feeding Practices among Kwun Tong Mothers. *J HK Med Assoc*, 1985; 37:181–84.
26. Davies, D. P. Nutritional Problems in Infancy and Early Childhood: A Commentary on the Contemporary Hong Kong Scene. *HK J Paediatr*, 1988; 5 (suppl.):135–51.
27. Leung, S.S.F. Auxological and Nutritional Status of Hong Kong Chinese Infants: Birth–Two Years. M.D. Thesis, The Chinese University of Hong Kong, 1990.
28. Davies, D. P., and Leung, S.S.F. Triceps and Subscapular Skinfold Growth from Birth to 18 Months in Hong Kong Chinese Infants. In Tanner, J. M., ed., *Perspectives in the Science of Growth and Development: Selected Papers from the Fifth International Auxology Congress.* London: Smith-Gordon and Company, 1989; 139–42.
29. Leung, S.S.F., Davies, D. P., Lui, S., *et al.* Iron Deficiency Is Uncommon in Healthy Infants at 18 Months. *J Trop Paed*, 1988; 34:100–3.
30. Leung, S.S.F., Lui, S., and Swaminathan, P. Vitamin D Status of Hong Kong Chinese Infants. *Acta Paed Scand*, 1989; 78:303–6.
31. Sung, R.Y.T., Lui, S., Lo, S., *et al.* Traditional Chinese Infant Supplementary Medical Foods Given by Mothers in Hong Kong. *Early Hum Dev*, 1988; 17:157–63.
32. Davies, D. P. The Importance of Genetic Influences on Growth in Early Childhood with Particular Reference to Children of Asiatic Origin. In

Waterlow, J., ed., *Linear Growth Retardation in Third World Countries*. Nestle Nutrition Workshop, No. 14. New York: Raven Press, Medical and Scientific Publishers, 1988.

33. Leung, S.S.F., Lui, S., and Davies, D. P. Cholesterol and Diet (letter). *Arch Dis Child*, 1989; 64:1,642–43.
34. Tarlow, M. J. Cholesterol and Diet. *Arch Dis Child*, 1989; 64:647–48.
35. Leung, D.T.Y., Tseng, R.Y.M., and Davies, D. P. Setting Up a Clinical Audit of Paediatric Morbidity in Hong Kong: Some Early Experiences. *Aust Paediatr J*, 1987; 23:111–13.
36. Tam, P.K.H., and Chan, J. Increasing Incidence of Hypertrophic Pyloric Stenosis. *Arch Dis Child*, 1991; 66:530–31.
37. Davies, D. P. Cot Death in Hong Kong: A Rare Problem. *Lancet*, 1985; 2:1,346–48.
38. Kelly, D. H., and Shannon, D. C. Sudden Infant Death Syndrome and Near Sudden Infant Death Syndrome: A Review of the Literature 1964 to 1982. *Pediatr Clin N Amer*, 1982; 29:1,241–61.
39. Lee, N.N.Y., Chan, Y. F., Davies, D. P., Lau, E., and Yip, D.C.P. Sudden Infant Death Syndrome in Hong Kong: Confirmation of Low Incidence. *BMJ*, 1989; 298:721.
40. Wigfield, R. E., Fleming, P. J., Beorg, P. J., Rudd, P. T., and Golding, J. Can the Fall in Avon's Sudden Death Rate Be Explained by Changes in Sleeping Position? *BMJ*, 1992; 304:282–83.
41. Mitchell, E. A., Stewart, A. W., Scragg, R., *et al.* Ethnic Differences in Mortality Rate from Sudden Infant Death Syndrome in New Zealand. *BMJ*, 1993; 306:13–16.
42. Balarajan, R., Raleigh, V. S., and Botting, B. Sudden Infant Death Syndrome and Post-natal Mortality in Immigrants in England and Wales. *BMJ*, 1989; 298:716–20.
43. Odent, M. Cot Deaths in Hong Kong (letter). *Lancet*, 1986; 1:214.
44. Grindulis, H., Scott, P. H., Belton, N. R., and Wharton, B. A. Combined Deficiency of Iron and Vitamin D in Asian Toddlers. *Arch Dis Child*, 1986; 61:843–48.
45. Mills, A. F. Surveillance for Anaemia: Risk Factors in Patterns of Milk Intake. *Arch Dis Child*, 1990; 65:428–31.
46. Wang, R.P.S., Chow, C. B., and Leung, N. K. Kawasaki Disease in Hong Kong. *HK J Paediatr*, 1986; 31:34–41.
47. Chan-Lui, W. Y., Lau, T.T.Y., and Leung, N. K. Myasthenia Gravis in Chinese Children. *Dev Med Child Neurol*, 1984; 26:717–24.
48. Hawkins, B. R., Yu, Y. L., Wong, V., *et al.* Possible Evidence for a Variant of Myasthenia Gravis Based on HLA Acetylcholine Receptor Antibody in Chinese Patients. *Q J Med*, 1989; 263:235 –41.

49. Sung, R.Y.T. Five Children with Drug Induced Extrapyramidal Symptoms. *HK J Paediatr*, 1985; 2:197–200.
50. Leung, D.T.Y., Tseng, R., Go, S. H., *et al.* Post-streptococcal Glomerulonephritis in Hong Kong. *Arch Dis Child*, 1987; 62:1,075–76.
51. Tsang, T. R., and Hut Saing. Endoscopic Diagnosis of Upper Gastro-intestinal Bleeding in Children. *HK J Paediatr*, 1988; 5:147–51.
52. Hopkinson, N. D. Systemic Lupus Erthematosus: Epidemiological Clues to Its Aetiology. *Br J Hosp Med*, 1991; 45:291–94.
53. Lau, Iris K. C., and Davies, D. P. Non-accidental Injury to Children in Hong Kong. *Welsh Paed J*, 1991; 3:10–14.
54. Hobbs, C. J., and Wynne, J. M. The Sexually Abused Battered Child. *Arch Dis Child*, 1990; 65:423–27.
55. Davies, D. P. Bedwetting in Hong Kong Chinese Children: A Relatively Uncommon Problem. *HK J Paediatr*, 1988; 1:65–66.
56. De Jonge, G. A. Epidemiology of Enuresis: A Survey of the Literature. In Kolvin, I., MacKeith, R. C., and Meadow, S. R., eds., *Bladder Control and Enuresis.* Clinics in Developmental Medicine, Nos. 48/49. London: Spastics International Medical Publications, William Heinemann Medical Books Ltd., 1973; 39–46.
57. Devlion, J. B., and O'Cathain, C. Predicting Treatment Outcome in Nocturnal Enuresis. *Arch Dis Child*, 1990; 65:1,158–61.
58. The Hong Kong Medical and Health Department, *Annual Report*, 1990.
59. The Hong Kong Medical and Health Department, *Annual Report*, 1989.
60. Tseng, R.Y.M., Lam, Y. M., and Davies, D. P. Hospitalization of Childhood Asthma in Hong Kong: 1976–1985. *Public Health*, 1988; 102:275–79.
61. Health Services in Hong Kong (editorial). *Lancet*, 1990; 1:666.
62. Davies, D. P. Health Services in Hong Kong (letter). *Lancet*, 1990; 1:666.
63. Field, C. E., and Baber, F. M. *Growing Up in Hong Kong*. Hong Kong: Hong Kong University Press, 1973.
64. Leung, S.S.F., Lam, Y. M., Lui, S., *et al.* Height, Weight and Head Circumference in Shatin Children 3–7 Years of Age: Further Evidence for Secular Change. *HK J Paediatr*, 1987; 4:43–51.
65. Lau, S. P., and Fung, K. P. Secular Trends of Growth in Hong Kong Children. *HK J Paediatr*, 1987; 4:33–42.